Mayo Clinic on Prostate Health

David M. Barrett, M.D.

Editor-in-Chief

MASON CREST PUBLISHERS

Philadelphia, Pennsylvania

Mayo Clinic on Prostate Health provides reliable, practical, easy-to-understand information on identifying and managing prostate conditions. Much of this information comes directly from the experience of urologists and other health care professionals at Mayo Clinic. This book supplements the advice of your physician, whom you should consult for individual medical problems. *Mayo Clinic on Prostate Health* does not endorse any company or product. Mayo, Mayo Clinic, and the Mayo triple-shield logo are registered marks of Mayo Foundation for Education and Research.

Hardcover Library Edition Published 2002
Mason Crest Publishers
370 Reed Road
Suite 302
Broomall, PA 19008-0914
(866) MCP-BOOK (toll free)

First printing

1 2 3 4 5 6 7 8 9 10

Library of Congress Cataloging-in-Publication Data on file at the Library of Congress

ISBN 1-59084-221-9

Photo credits: cover photos and pages 1, 23, 57, 135 from PhotoDisc.

Printed in the United States of America

About Prostate Disease

Odds are that during your lifetime, you'll experience a prostate problem. Prostate disease affects more than half of all men and becomes more prevalent with age. Inflammation, enlargement and cancer of the prostate gland are three typical problems men face. Although annoying and sometimes painful, inflammation and enlargement generally aren't life-threatening. Prostate cancer, on the other hand, is now the most common cancer in men and the second highest cause of cancer deaths in men. However, with early diagnosis, it can often be successfully treated.

Within these pages you'll find practical advice you can use to identify and treat prostate problems before they become difficult to manage or a threat to your life. You'll also learn about lifestyle changes that may reduce your risk of prostate disease. This book is based on the expertise of Mayo Clinic doctors and the advice they give day in and day out in caring for their patients.

About Mayo Clinic

Mayo Clinic evolved from the frontier practice of Dr. William Worrall Mayo, and the partnership of his two sons, William J. and Charles H. Mayo, in the early 1900s. Pressed by the demands of their busy surgical practice in Rochester, Minn., the Mayo brothers invited other physicians to join them, pioneering the private group practice of medicine. Today, with more than 2,000 physicians and scientists at its three major locations in Rochester, Minn., Jacksonville, Fla., and Scottsdale, Ariz., Mayo Clinic is dedicated to providing comprehensive diagnosis, accurate answers and effective treatments.

With its depth of knowledge, experience and expertise, Mayo Clinic occupies an unparalleled position as a health information resource. Since 1983, Mayo Clinic has published reliable health information for millions of consumers through award-winning newsletters, books and online services. Revenue from the publishing activities supports Mayo Clinic programs, including medical education and research.

Editorial Staff

Editor in Chief
David M. Barrett, M.D.

Medical Editors
Michael L. Blute, M.D.
Reza S. Malek, M.D.

Senior Editor
N. Nicole Spelhaug

Managing Editor
Karen R. Wallevand

Copy Editor
Edith Schwager

Editorial Researcher
Brian M. Laing

Contributing Writers
Rebecca Gonzalez-Campoy
Lynn Madsen
D. R. Martin
Stephen M. Miller
Catherine Stroebel
Susan Wichmann

Creative Director
Daniel W. Brevick

Graphic Designer
Kathryn K. Shepel

**Layout and
Production Artist**
Stewart J. Koski

Medical Illustrators
Brian S. Fyffe
Steven P. Graepel
John V. Hagen
Craig R. King
M. Alice McKinney
James D. Postier

Secretarial Assistant
Kathleen K. Iverson

Indexer
Larry Harrison

Reviewers and Additional Contributors

Jon B. Closson, M.D
Edward T. Creagan, M.D.
Kelli C. Fee-Schroeder, R.N.
Renee E. Kromrey, R.N.
Jennifer K. Nelson, R.D.

Preface

Prostate disease is, in essence, the male counterpart of breast disease. Just as women fear breast cancer, men worry about their prostates. That's understandable. Prostate cancer is now the most common cancer in men. Like breast cancer in women, treatment for prostate cancer can sometimes lead to difficult decisions and unexpected consequences.

But there's more to this story that you should know, and that's why we wrote this book. Prostate conditions — even cancer — are often easily treated. The key to a good outcome is early diagnosis. When detected early, cancer and other prostate disorders have the best chance of successful treatment with minimal side effects. That's why it's important that you know the early warning signs of prostate disease and, if you're at least 40 years old, that you have a yearly prostate checkup.

In this book, you'll find information on what to expect during a typical prostate checkup. We discuss the prostate-specific antigen (PSA) screening test and Mayo Clinic urologists' view of the test. We explain three common prostate disorders, symptoms that ordinarily accompany each, and various treatment options. To help you determine the best form of treatment, we identify factors to consider and questions to ask your doctor. We devote an entire chapter to potential side effects of prostate cancer treatment and how to manage those problems. We give you information on ways you may be able to reduce your risk of prostate disease with diet and exercise. You'll also find answers to commonly asked questions.

We believe that the more you know about prostate disease and the factors that affect it, the greater are your chances of identifying problems early and making good decisions regarding treatment. Along with the advice of your physician, this book can help you live a longer, healthier life.

David M. Barrett, M.D.
Editor in Chief

Contents

Part 3: Prostate Cancer

Part 4: Prostate Health

Part 1

Prostate Primer

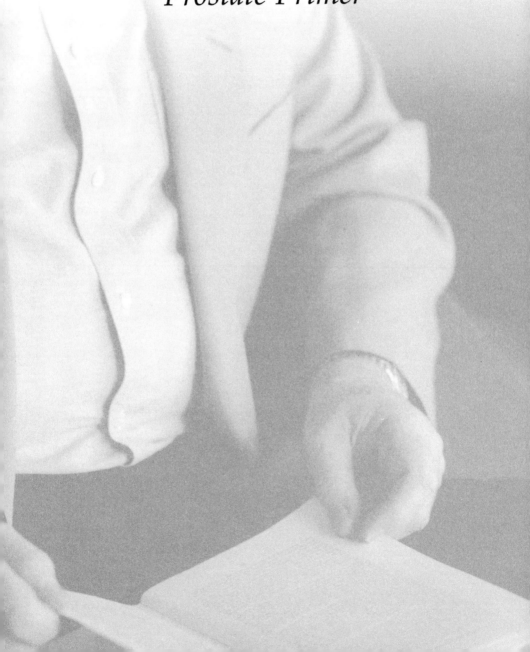

Chapter 1

About the Prostate

Prostate disease is one of the most common health problems men face, and prostate cancer is among the most feared. That's because prostate cancer, like breast cancer, often strikes at the core of human sexuality. Beyond the fear of cancer itself are the possible consequences of treatment — bladder control problems (incontinence) and an inability to achieve an erection (impotence). These conditions can be as difficult as the cancer, shattering confidence and evoking feelings of lost masculinity.

But there's no need to live in fear. If caught early, prostate cancer often can be successfully treated. Improved surgical techniques are reducing the risks of impotence and incontinence. And when these conditions do occur, various treatments may limit their effects.

It's also important to understand that cancer isn't the source of all prostate problems. Inflammation and benign enlargement of the prostate are equally common conditions. Unlike cancer, these problems generally aren't life-threatening, but without early and proper treatment, they can become irritating, debilitating and painful.

For many men, prostate disease is a fact of life that comes with age. However, by getting regular checkups and working with your doctor, you can reduce your risk of serious disease and keep your condition from seriously interfering with your routine. This book can help you better understand why prostate problems occur, identify symptoms early, and make informed decisions regarding treatment.

A healthy prostate

Found only in men, the prostate gland surrounds the bottom portion ("neck") of the bladder. It's located behind the pubic bone and in front of the rectum. About the size and shape of a walnut, the prostate is made up of smooth muscle, spongy tissue, and tiny ducts and glands, and is covered by a thin membrane called the capsule.

At birth, the prostate is about the size of a pea. It continues to grow until about age 20, when it reaches normal adult size. It remains that size until about age 45, when it often begins to grow again.

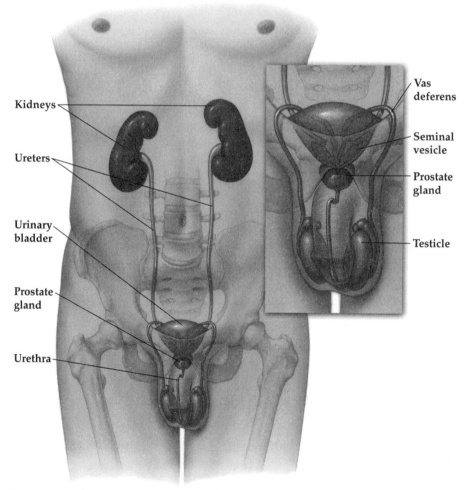

The prostate gland is located deep within the pelvis, just below the bladder. It affects the health of both the reproductive and the urinary systems.

Reproductive system

The prostate's primary function is to produce most of the fluids in semen, the fluid that transports sperm. Tiny ducts within your prostate convey this fluid to the urethra, the channel that drains fluid from the bladder and out through the penis.

During orgasm, prostate fluid mixes with fluid from the seminal vesicles, located on each side of the prostate, and with sperm to form semen. Sperm travel up from your testicles through long tubes called the vasa deferentia (VAY-zuh DEF-ur-EN-shuh). Muscle contractions cause ejaculation, in which the semen is propelled through the urethra and out of the penis.

To make sure semen doesn't move in the wrong direction and back up into the bladder, a ring of muscle at the neck of the bladder (internal sphincter) remains tightened during ejaculation. The sphincter also keeps urine from discharging with the semen.

Urinary system

The prostate gland isn't a primary component of the urinary system, but because of its location, it's also important to your urinary health.

Your urinary system begins with your kidneys, which cleanse body fluids and produce urine. Urine travels from your kidneys to your bladder through long muscular tubes called ureters (you-REE-ters). Your bladder stores the urine until you urinate. During urination, urine exits your bladder through the urethra.

Your prostate gland surrounds the top portion of the urethra. Think of your prostate as a small apple with its core missing. The urethra runs through the missing core. When your prostate is healthy, this doesn't pose any problems. But if disease develops in the prostate, tissue in this gland can swell or grow, squeezing the urethra and affecting your ability to urinate.

When things go wrong

You aren't destined to develop prostate disease. Some men go through life without any prostate problems. Many, however, aren't so lucky. By the time they reach their senior years, a large number of men experience some type of prostate problem. Symptoms may range from minor and mildly annoying to serious and painful.

Three types of diseases can affect the prostate gland. Often, but not always, they occur at different periods in a man's life.

Inflammation

With this condition, your prostate swells and becomes tender. Many times, a bacterial infection is the source of the inflammation. Other times, the cause is unknown. Called prostatitis (PROS-tuh-TIE-tis), prostate inflammation is typically most common between ages 25 and 45.

Noncancerous enlargement

Around age 45, tissue inside the prostate gland often begins to grow again. This growth is called benign prostatic hyperplasia (pros-TAT-ik HY-pur-PLAY-zhuh), or BPH. It typically occurs in the center portion of the gland, causing prostate tissue to press on the urethra and produce urinary problems. Many men first experience symptoms between ages 55 and 60. Others don't have symptoms until their 70s or 80s.

Cancer

Prostate cancer is most common after age 50. It increases in frequency as men get older. Prostate cancer results from abnormal and uncontrolled growth of tissue cells. Unlike BPH, in which most of the growth is in the innermost region of the gland, with prostate cancer, tumors generally develop in the outer portion of the prostate. Depending on the type of cancer, these tumors may grow very slowly or at a more rapid pace.

Symptoms that may signal a problem

Irritating or painful symptoms will often alert you to a prostate problem. This is especially true for prostate inflammation or enlargement.

The following symptoms are often associated with prostate disease. However, they aren't limited to the prostate. Other conditions, such as a urinary infection or kidney stones, can produce some of the same symptoms:

- Difficulty starting your urine stream
- Decreased strength and force of your urine stream
- Urinating more frequently
- Feeling as if your bladder isn't empty, even after you've just urinated
- Dribbling after you've finished urinating
- An urgent need to urinate
- Blood in the urine
- Painful ejaculation
- Pain or a burning sensation while urinating
- Tenderness or pain in the pelvis
- Persistent back or hip pain
- Pain or swelling in the testicles

Unfortunately, prostate cancer produces few, if any, symptoms in its early stages. It's not until later, when the disease is more difficult to treat, that symptoms such as urination difficulties or back pain may develop. That's why it's important to have regular prostate checkups to catch the disease early.

Are you at risk?

There's no simple formula to tell precisely who will encounter prostate problems. However, various factors — some of them controllable, some not — can increase your odds.

Uncontrollable risk factors

These are the most common risk factors for prostate disease:

Age. As you get older, your risk of BPH and prostate cancer increases. More than half of men older than age 50, and 80 percent of men in their 70s, experience prostate enlargement. In addition, more than 80 percent of men with a diagnosis of prostate cancer are older than age 65.

Ethnic group. For reasons that aren't well understood, black men are more likely to have prostate cancer than men of any other group. They're also more likely to have cancer at a younger age, and to have an aggressive form of prostate cancer. Asian men, on the other hand, have the lowest rate of prostate cancer. The rate of prostate cancer in Hispanic and American Indian men is lower than in whites.

Family history. Studies show that if your father or brother has prostate cancer, your risk of the disease is about twice as great as that of the average American male. And depending on the number of relatives with prostate cancer and the age at which they had it, your risk could be even higher. In families with a history of prostate cancer, the cancer generally strikes at a younger age.

Family history also may play a role in risk of BPH. Age is the primary risk factor for the condition. But among men who have BPH in their 40s or early 50s, many carry an inherited gene that predisposes them to the disease. Carrying the gene doesn't mean that disease is inevitable. It simply increases the risk.

Controllable risk factors

Risk of prostate cancer differs among populations. Because these differences don't appear to be genetic, researchers suspect that environment and lifestyle factors may play a role in your risk of prostate disease. However, at this point, there are more questions regarding what these factors might be than there are answers.

Environment. Researchers are studying whether occupational exposure to certain substances may play an important role. Higher death rates from prostate cancer can be found in certain blue-collar workers, such as farmers, mechanics, welders and industrial employees, than in men in other occupations.

A 1999 Mayo Clinic study of more than 1,000 Iowa farmers found that those age 70 and older are twice as likely to have prostate cancer as nonfarmers the same age. The study also suggests that the increase may be due to occupational exposure and not dietary or lifestyle factors.

Diet. There's some evidence that a high-fat diet may increase the risk of prostate cancer. Researchers at the Harvard Medical School and the Harvard School of Public Health evaluated the diets of more than 50,000 health professionals for 4 years. They found that the men with high-fat diets were nearly twice as likely to have prostate cancer as men who ate less fat.

Researchers theorize that the increased risk may be because fat increases production of the hormone testosterone, which in turn speeds development of prostate cancer cells. If this theory proves correct, you may be able to reduce your risk of prostate cancer, or slow its development, by limiting fat in your diet.

There's also evidence that chemicals found in soy products and certain vegetables and fruits may lower your risk of prostate cancer. Later in this book (page 137), we look at different ways you may be able to protect yourself against prostate disease or delay its development, including eating healthy foods.

Supplemental hormones. Large doses of the nutritional supplement dehydroepiandrosterone (DHEA) may aggravate BPH or promote development of prostate cancer. DHEA is a hormone that occurs naturally in your body. It's thought to be a precursor hormone that's easily converted into other hormones, such as testosterone and estrogen. DHEA levels in your body increase sharply at puberty, peak during adulthood, and then decrease gradually as you age.

DHEA supplements are promoted to slow aging, burn fat, build muscle and strengthen the immune system. They're also touted as a treatment for various illnesses, including Alzheimer's disease and Parkinson's disease. Studies so far haven't proven that the supplements provide benefits. Their long-term effects and how they may interact with other drugs also are uncertain.

Answers to your questions

Is it possible to be born with an abnormal prostate gland?
Yes. You can have a congenital abnormality in your prostate. Because of the location where the prostate develops, men with congenital prostate abnormalities sometimes also have kidney abnormalities. These conditions aren't common, however, and they

can easily be ruled out through X-ray or ultrasound images of the prostate gland and the kidneys.

I once had a sexually transmitted disease. Does this increase my risk of prostate problems?
Possibly. Some sexually transmitted diseases, such as gonorrhea and a chlamydia infection, may cause inflammation in your urethra, the tube that carries urine out of your bladder. This inflammation can sometimes produce scar tissue that can narrow or block the urethra, increasing your risk of urinary infections or infection in your prostate gland (prostatitis).

Is it true that a vasectomy can increase my risk of prostate cancer?
No. A few studies raised speculation that having a vasectomy may increase the risk of prostate cancer. However, researchers with the National Institutes of Health have reviewed all of the data on vasectomies. They concluded that the sterilization procedure doesn't increase a man's risk of getting prostate cancer.

Researchers believe that the questions raised in the studies can be explained by the fact that most vasectomies are done by urologists, and that men who have a good relationship with a urologist are more likely to get regular prostate checkups. Therefore, their cancer is detected earlier than in men who don't get regular prostate examinations.

Chapter 2

Getting a Prostate Checkup

You are your own best weapon against prostate disease. If you can catch the condition in its early stages, you have a good chance of successful treatment. How do you do that? With regular prostate checkups.

There's no specific schedule for when you should have prostate checkups. If you're in your 20s or 30s, a yearly exam generally isn't necessary, unless you have a strong family history of prostate disease or you're experiencing prostate-related symptoms.

Once you reach your 40s, however, you should have a prostate examination yearly and continue to have regular checkups throughout your lifetime. What's involved in a typical exam will vary, depending on your age, doctor, family history and test results.

Basic diagnostic tests

Most men have a prostate checkup in conjunction with their yearly physical examination. In addition to standard procedures and tests that go along with a physical exam, such as checking your blood pressure and listening to your lungs, you may have some or all of the following:

Digital rectal exam (DRE)
This is a basic and easy screening test for prostate disease. However,

it may well rank among the most anxious aspects of a physical exam for many men because it seems embarrassing or they find it uncomfortable.

To perform the exam, your doctor puts on an examination glove and applies a lubricant to one finger. You're then asked to bend over — perhaps leaning on an examination table — while your doctor gently inserts the lubricated finger into your rectum.

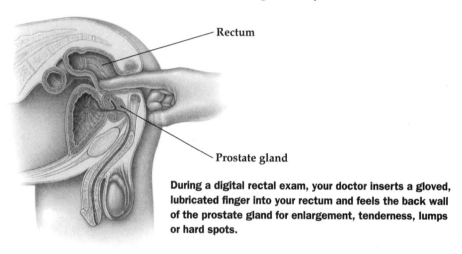

Rectum

Prostate gland

During a digital rectal exam, your doctor inserts a gloved, lubricated finger into your rectum and feels the back wall of the prostate gland for enlargement, tenderness, lumps or hard spots.

Because the prostate gland is located adjacent to the rectum, your doctor can feel the back wall of the gland with his or her finger. A gland that feels enlarged may indicate benign prostatic hyperplasia (BPH). If the gland feels tender to the touch, it may be a sign of prostatitis. In addition, the outer portion of the gland is where about 70 percent of cancerous tumors develop. In their early stages, they often feel like nodules or hard spots. If your doctor detects such an abnormality, it doesn't necessarily mean you have cancer, but he or she will want to perform additional tests. Other conditions, including a prostate infection or formation of small stones in the gland, can produce similar characteristics.

A recent Mayo Clinic study found strong evidence that men who didn't receive regular digital rectal exams were more likely to die of prostate cancer than a similar group of men who did have regular exams. The researchers believe that timely digital rectal exams could have saved the lives of 50 percent to 70 percent of these men.

There are differing opinions among health care organizations as to when men should begin having a digital rectal exam. Some groups recommend age 50, others age 40. Mayo Clinic urologists agree with the recommendation of the American Urological Association (AUA) that you have a yearly DRE beginning at age 40.

Urine test

This test looks for abnormalities in your urine that may indicate a problem. If your urine contains more white blood cells than normal, you may have an infection in your prostate gland or urinary tract.

Red blood cells in your urine may signal inflammation of the prostate or, perhaps, a tumor. Other conditions, including inflammation of the urethra or bladder problems, also can produce blood in your urine.

In addition, if your doctor thinks you have BPH, a urine test result that's normal can help confirm his or her diagnosis.

Blood test

A small amount of blood is drawn from your arm and analyzed for a substance called prostate-specific antigen (PSA). The antigen is naturally produced in your prostate gland to help liquefy semen. A small amount of it, however, enters your bloodstream and circulates in your blood. If higher than normal levels of PSA are detected in your blood, it could indicate prostate inflammation, enlargement or cancer.

Most men first have a PSA test between the ages of 40 and 50. In the next sections, we discuss this test in detail and the controversy surrounding it.

Ultrasound

If your doctor has some concerns about the results of your digital rectal exam or urine or blood tests, he or she may want to take a closer look at your prostate. This can be done with a procedure called a transrectal ultrasound.

Ultrasonography is an imaging technique that uses sound waves to see inside your body. Ultrasound operates like radar, sending out sound waves that are reflected or absorbed to varying degrees, depending on the consistency of an object. Because cancerous tissue is thicker and more dense than healthy tissue, the sound wave reflections are different.

During a transrectal ultrasound test, your doctor inserts a small, lubricated probe, which emits sound waves, into your rectum. The reflections from the waves are translated by a computer and converted into a video picture. The procedure is harmless, although some men find it a little uncomfortable.

If your doctor doesn't find anything serious, you may not need further tests. If the ultrasound result suggests cancer, a biopsy is needed to confirm its presence.

More on the prostate-specific antigen (PSA) test

The PSA test was approved by the Food and Drug Administration in 1986 as a means to help detect prostate cancer. Since the test was approved, there's been an increase in the number of cases of the disease — often in its early stages, when the cancer can be cured.

After a blood sample is taken from your arm, the sample is sent to a laboratory where it's tested with a procedure called an immunochemical assay. This test determines how much prostate-specific antigen is circulating in your blood.

A reading between 0 and 4 nanograms per milliliter (ng/mL) is normal. However, because PSA levels tend to increase with a person's age, some medical centers have adjusted their standards based on age (see "Mayo Clinic PSA standards").

If your PSA level is above normal, that doesn't necessarily mean you have cancer. Some men have higher than normal PSA levels and healthy prostates. Conditions other than cancer can increase the amount of PSA circulating in your blood.

BPH. Noncancerous enlargement of the prostate is the most common condition that can lead to an elevated PSA reading. As prostate tissues grow, cells within the tissue produce more PSA than normal — sometimes up to three times higher than normal.

Mayo Clinic PSA standards

Mayo Clinic urologists use the following age-adjusted scale to determine a normal PSA range, based on the test used at Mayo.

Age	Normal PSA Range
40 to 49	0 to 2.5 ng/mL*
50 to 59	0 to 3.5 ng/mL
60 to 69	0 to 4.5 ng/mL
✳ 70 to 79	0 to 6.5 ng/mL

* Nanograms per milliliter

Prostatitis. Irritation of the prostate due to inflammation or an infection can cause cells in the gland to release increased amounts of PSA.

Cancer. Cancerous cells in the prostate also produce PSA. A higher than normal PSA reading may indicate the presence of cancer in prostate tissues.

Other factors also can increase your PSA level:

Ejaculation. As you get older, your prostate gland is more likely to leak PSA into your bloodstream during orgasm. Men ages 50 to 80 can experience a 40 percent increase in the amount of PSA in their blood less than an hour after ejaculation. This increase can continue for up to 48 hours. That means you should abstain from sexual activity for at least 2 days before a PSA test to help ensure accurate results.

Urinary tract infection. Like an infection in your prostate gland, a urinary tract infection can increase your PSA level.

Recent prostate procedures. These procedures, discussed more fully later in the book, can temporarily irritate your prostate gland, producing inflammation and above-normal levels of PSA:

- Prostate biopsy
- Transurethral resection of the prostate
- Transurethral incision of the prostate
- Prostate "massage"
- Microwave therapy of the prostate
- Laser therapy of the prostate
- Balloon dilation of the prostate

After having one of these procedures, you should wait from 2 weeks up to 2 months to have a PSA test. This allows your PSA to return to the level where it was just before the procedure.

How accurate is the PSA test?

The PSA test detects cancer in its early stages about 80 percent of the time. In about 20 percent of men with early prostate cancer, the results come back normal. This is one drawback of the test — in 1 out of 5 men with prostate cancer it may not catch the cancer early.

Another drawback of the PSA test is that it can't distinguish between cancer and other prostate diseases. Among men with an elevated PSA level, only one-third have cancer. Increased PSA levels in the other two-thirds may be the result of BPH, prostatitis

---

Finasteride and PSA

Finasteride (Proscar) is a medication used to treat BPH. It shrinks the prostate gland by suppressing certain hormones that stimulate prostate growth. Finasteride is the same drug taken to promote hair growth in balding men, sold under the brand name Propecia.

By altering the level of hormones in the prostate gland, finasteride reduces production of PSA in the gland. The decrease in PSA can be as much as 50 percent and can occur even if you have prostate cancer. Instead of going up to signal the presence of cancer, your PSA goes down.

This raises a question regarding the accuracy of PSA testing in men who use the medication. Some doctors believe PSA tests aren't beneficial for men taking finasteride. Others, however, believe that by reducing normal PSA ranges in men taking finasteride, the PSA test can still be useful. For example, if the normal PSA range for a 70-year-old man is 0 to 6.5 ng/mL, the normal range for a 70-year-old man taking finasteride would be 0 to 3.25 ng/mL.

It's essential for your doctor to be aware if you're taking the medication so he or she can monitor and interpret the PSA results appropriately.

or some other factor. As a result, many men who don't have cancer must undergo additional tests to rule out cancer.

Still, the PSA test is a more accurate screening test than, for example, mammography for breast cancer or a chest X-ray for lung cancer.

The great debate

Not all doctors and medical organizations agree that the benefits of the PSA test outweigh its limitations. That is why this simple test has become one of the most controversial screening tools in medicine today.

Its benefits

There's little doubt that regular PSA screening can help identify prostate cancer long before any symptoms become apparent. The PSA test is often able to detect cancer when it's still confined to the prostate gland. Localized cancer is much easier to treat and cure than cancer that has spread to other organs.

Not all prostate cancers are alike. Some grow very slowly and remain within the prostate gland. Others are more aggressive and can spread rather quickly to other organs. If your PSA test detects what turns out to be an aggressive form of prostate cancer, it could literally be a lifesaver.

The year 1997 marked the first-ever reduction in deaths from prostate cancer. Many doctors believe the PSA test is a major factor behind the decrease. However, health experts haven't been able to prove with certainty that the screening test reduces prostate cancer deaths.

Its limitations

The PSA test is far from ideal or perfect. In the 20 percent of men in whom the test fails to identify prostate cancer, it may give them a false sense of security about their prostate health. And among men with an elevated PSA, two out of three often go through needless worry and unnecessary, expensive medical procedures.

There's also a question of whether the test leads to needless treatment. If you have a slow-growing cancer, you may be able to live with it for years without its causing any problems. But for some men, this can be difficult to accept. When they learn they have cancer, they want to do something to get rid of it, such as undergo surgery or radiation. These treatments may produce side effects, including incontinence or impotence. The result can be a decrease in the quality of life for men who could otherwise live healthy, productive lives.

Finally, there's the issue of whether early detection of prostate cancer actually saves lives. Certain studies, including some at Mayo Clinic, contend it does. Other studies, however, aren't so supportive. They show that in some parts of the country prostate cancer deaths haven't decreased at all since PSA screening became available. One reason for the difference in findings may be that in some areas the test has been available for only a few years, and it may take more time to substantiate its life-saving benefits.

A future settlement?

Two studies now under way may provide some answers and help settle the PSA debate. However, it will be years before the results are known.

PLCO. The Prostate, Lung, Colorectal, and Ovarian trial is a large, multimillion-dollar study sponsored by the National Cancer Institute to determine whether screening and early detection of cancer save lives. For prostate cancer, men are screened once a year for 4 years and then followed for 12 more years.

PIVOT. The Prostate cancer Intervention Versus Observatory Trial is funded by the Department of Veterans Affairs and the National Cancer Institute.

PIVOT is another large, lengthy study that hopes to determine the best way to treat cancer confined to the prostate gland — whether to perform surgery to remove the gland or let the gland alone and watch to see if the cancer spreads ("watchful waiting"). Participants in the study have regular examinations and periodically fill out questionnaires regarding their quality of life.

Current recommendations

So, in the meantime, what do you do? Should you have a PSA test or not?

There's no definitive answer. Of the medical organizations that have taken a stand on the PSA test, about one-third support its use, one-third are neutral, and one-third don't support it.

The American Cancer Society (ACS) and the AUA are among its supporters. They recommend that the PSA test be offered to all men beginning at age 50, along with information on the benefits and risks should cancer be found. They also recommend that black men and others with a family history of prostate cancer begin PSA screening at age 40.

As for how long you should continue to take the test, the ACS and AUA recommend lifelong screening. Some doctors, however, feel that after age 70 the test begins to lose its value and may no longer be necessary.

Mayo Clinic's view

Mayo Clinic urologists understand the pitfalls of the PSA test and agree that it's far from perfect. But they support its use because it's the best screening tool available for detecting prostate cancer in its early stages. It's especially beneficial for younger men who have curable cancers.

As with all other cancers, the earlier prostate cancer is found, the greater your chance for a complete recovery. Early detection also allows time to make good treatment decisions.

In accordance with the ACS and AUA, Mayo Clinic urologists recommend an annual PSA test beginning at age 50, unless you're at high risk of prostate cancer. If you're black or you have a family history of prostate cancer you may want to begin at age 40. Mayo Clinic urologists also recommend that you continue to have yearly PSA tests until age 75. Beyond age 75, a yearly digital rectal exam is often sufficient.

If you have concerns about the PSA test — your chances of getting a false result or what you should do if cancer is found — don't hesitate to discuss these concerns with your doctor beforehand.

In search of a better screening tool

Researchers continue to look for a more accurate and specific screening test for prostate cancer that can reduce or eliminate some disadvantages of the PSA test. Several options are currently under study:

Free-PSA test. PSA comes in two forms — PSA that's bound by blood proteins and PSA that's unbound, called "free" PSA. The current test measures both bound and unbound PSA to determine the total amount of PSA in your blood. Researchers have learned, however, that cancer is more likely to produce bound PSA, whereas BPH is linked to an increase in free PSA.

The free-PSA test indicates how much PSA circulates alone in blood and how much is bound together with blood proteins. The lower the percentage of free PSA, the more likely that cancer may be responsible for the increase in your PSA level. The higher the percentage of free PSA, the greater the chance BPH may be the cause.

PSA velocity test. This test charts the rate of change in your PSA levels. Scientists believe that the number of PSA molecules grows more quickly in someone who has prostate cancer rather than BPH or prostatitis.

PSA density test. Prostate-specific antigen density (PSAD) is determined by dividing your PSA level by your prostate volume. Your PSA volume can be obtained by ultrasound. A higher PSAD generally indicates a greater likelihood of cancer.

Ultrasensitive PSA test. This specialized test is capable of detecting minute quantities of PSA in your bloodstream. If you've already been treated for prostate cancer, it may detect a recurrence of cancer far earlier than is possible with other tests — perhaps by 1 or 2 years.

Other markers. A number of other substances similar to PSA may serve as markers for early prostate cancer. They include human glandular kallikrein, chromogranin A, and prostate-specific membrane antigen (PSMA). These screening tests could eventually prove to be a more reliable indicator of prostate cancer.

Gene research. If researchers can identify a gene responsible for prostate cancer, men who carry this gene could be monitored more closely to identify cancer in its very early stages. These men may even be able to prevent cancer through lifestyle changes, including a change in diet.

Answers to your questions

Can my family physician do a prostate examination?
Absolutely. Family physicians are vital to the process of screening men for prostate cancer or other abnormalities. The digital rectal exam and PSA tests are routine tests that virtually every family doctor is familiar with.

When should I see a urologist?
Your family physician may recommend that you see a urologist if he or she has questions regarding your test results, suspects prostate cancer, or believes that a urologist could better treat noncancerous conditions, such as BPH or prostatitis. If you have a problem urinating, your PSA level is elevated, or your family doctor finds an abnormality during a digital rectal examination, it may be advisable to see a urologist.

Can I request a PSA test if my doctor doesn't routinely give me one?
You can. Most health plans allow you to obtain the medical tests you desire. However, the plan may not pay for the test. Check with your doctor and your insurance provider to clarify if a PSA test is covered by your insurance plan before requesting the test. If you have to pay for it yourself, a PSA test usually costs about $45.

My PSA level has always been very low. It's still within the normal range, but it has increased. Should I be concerned?
As you age, your PSA level may increase slightly. However, a noticeable change in your PSA should be followed with a thorough evaluation, even if the reading is "normal."

I'm 79 years old. Why don't I need a PSA screening test anymore?
PSA tests are most beneficial for detecting cancer in its very early
stages. If you have early signs of prostate cancer after age 75, it's
unlikely that the cancer will cause serious difficulty. Therefore,
there's no need to put you through unnecessary testing and the
worry that can accompany cancer. Men who develop prostate
cancer late in life generally die of causes other than their cancer.

Part 2

Noncancerous Conditions

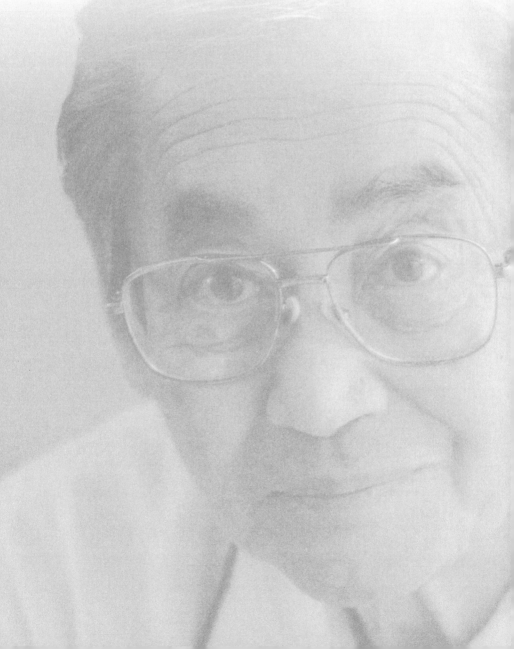

Chapter 3

Living with Prostatitis

One of the most common prostate problems men encounter is one you seldom hear about. According to some estimates, up to a quarter of all visits men make to a doctor for genital or urinary problems are related to prostatitis. Not only is this condition common, it can be both tough to diagnose and difficult to treat.

Prostatitis is a general term for inflammation of the prostate gland. The inflammation may be due to an infection or another factor that's irritating the gland. Although many things are unclear about the disease, doctors have found that an accurate diagnosis is crucial to treating it. That's because prostatitis can emerge in at least three forms:

Acute bacterial
This is the least common and most severe form of the disease. It results from an infection in the prostate gland that produces severe and often sudden symptoms. These may include a combination of:
- Fever
- Chills
- A general flulike feeling
- Pain in the lower back and genital area
- Pain or a burning sensation when urinating
- Inability to urinate or decreased urine flow
- Inability to empty the bladder during urination

- A frequent and sometimes urgent need to urinate
- Blood-tinged urine
- Painful ejaculation

Bacteria commonly found in the urinary tract or large intestine are most often responsible for this type of prostatitis. Because acute bacterial prostatitis can lead to serious problems, including an inability to urinate and infection in the bloodstream (bacteremia), it's important that you see a doctor right away. If your symptoms are severe, you may need to be hospitalized for a few days until they begin to improve.

Chronic bacterial

This condition also is caused by a bacterial infection. However, unlike acute prostatitis, symptoms typically develop more slowly and they're often less severe. They may include:

- Frequent urination
- A sudden or compelling urge to urinate
- Pain or a burning sensation when urinating
- Excessive nighttime urination
- Pain in the lower back and genital area
- Difficulty starting or continuing urination
- A diminished urine flow
- Occasional blood in semen
- Painful ejaculation
- Slight fever
- Recurring bladder infection

What causes a chronic bacterial infection isn't certain. Like an acute infection, it may result from bacteria in your urinary tract. Other causes may include a bladder or blood infection. The infection may follow trauma to your urinary tract or insertion of an instrument — usually a catheter — into your urethra. That's why some doctors routinely prescribe antibiotics after use of a urinary catheter.

Sometimes calcified stones can form in your prostate gland and attract bacteria. Rarely, the infection results from an underlying structural defect in your prostate that becomes a collection site for bacteria.

This form of prostatitis is often ongoing (chronic) because the infection can be difficult to get rid of. Antibiotics taken to kill the bacteria have a difficult time penetrating prostate tissues.

Chronic nonbacterial

Most men with prostatitis have this type. Unfortunately, it's also the most difficult to diagnose and treat. Instead of trying to cure the disease, the main goal of treatment is usually to find relief from its symptoms.

Symptoms of chronic nonbacterial prostatitis are about the same as those for chronic bacterial prostatitis. But one distinguishing factor separates the two: In this kind of prostatitis, your doctor isn't able to detect bacteria in your urine or in fluid from your prostate gland. However, white blood cells in urine specimens signal the presence of inflammation.

The main reason nonbacterial prostatitis is so difficult to diagnose and treat is that its cause is unknown. Theories abound as to possible triggers of the inflammation. However, none are certain and many aren't well understood. Among the possible causes are:

Sexual activity. Sexually active younger men with inflammation of the urethra (urethritis) or a sexually transmitted disease, such as gonorrhea or a chlamydia infection, are more likely to develop chronic nonbacterial prostatitis. In some men, a reduction in the frequency of sexual intercourse also may be a contributing factor.

Other infectious agents. The inflammation may be related to some kind of infectious agent current techniques can't detect.

Anxiety or stress. These conditions may cause you to tighten the urinary sphincter muscle, which controls urine flow from the bladder, and those muscles located between your legs that support the bladder and rectum (pelvic floor muscles). Muscle tightening may prevent the muscles from relaxing properly, and may irritate the gland or cause fluids in the urethra to back up into your prostate, irritating inner tissues.

Stop-and-start urination. Instead of relaxing and letting urine flow freely, some men frequently stop and start while urinating. Stopping urine flow may cause urine in the urethra to back up into, and irritate, the prostate.

Heavy lifting. Lifting heavy objects while your bladder is full also may cause urine to back up and seep into your prostate.

Certain occupations. Occupations that subject the prostate to a great deal of vibration, such as truck driving or riding on heavy equipment, may be associated with chronic bacterial infection.

Recreational activities. Frequent activities such as bicycling or jogging may possibly irritate the gland.

What kind do you have?

The two most important steps in diagnosing prostatitis are ruling out other conditions that can cause similar symptoms and determining the type of prostatitis you have.

To do this, your doctor will ask you questions about your symptoms: What are they? Do they come and go, or are they persistent? When did they first occur? Can you recall any changes in your routine or lifestyle about the time they began? Your doctor may also ask you about recent medical procedures, previous infections, your sexual habits, your occupation, and whether you have a family history of prostate problems.

A physical examination generally follows. It may include checking your abdomen and pelvic area for unusual tenderness, and a digital rectal exam of your prostate gland. An inflamed prostate often feels enlarged and tender to the touch.

During the digital exam, your doctor may collect fluid from your prostate gland. To do this, he or she will rub rather vigorously against the gland with a gloved finger, forcing fluid out of the gland and into your urethra. From there it passes through your penis. The fluid is collected and examined under a microscope for signs of an infection or inflammation. This procedure is often referred to as prostate "massage" or prostate "stripping."

A urine sample also is necessary to check for bacteria and white blood cells. White blood cells indicate inflammation. Bacteria point to an infection. If your urine tests positive for both — inflammation and infection — you likely have bacterial prostatitis. If the test finds white blood cells but no bacteria, then you probably have the nonbacterial form. If neither bacteria nor white blood cells are found, your symptoms may be related to other disorders. These could include a condition called prostatodynia, discussed later in this chapter.

Designing a treatment plan

Once your doctor determines the kind of prostatitis you have, the two of you can work together on a plan for treating the condition, and possibly curing it. Since the cause of chronic nonbacterial prostatitis is often unknown, this form of the disease can be difficult to cure. However, with some patience and experimentation, many men find ways to manage the condition and keep it from interfering seriously with their daily lives.

Medications
One or more of the following drugs may help cure or control your symptoms:

Antibiotics. Antibiotics are a traditional first line of treatment for all forms of prostatitis. Your doctor will likely start you off on a drug that fights a broad spectrum of bacteria. Once the specific type of bacterium that's causing your infection has been determined — based on your urine and prostatic fluid samples — you may have a different drug prescribed that's more effective at killing the bacteria.

How long you'll need to take an antibiotic will vary depending on how well your infection responds to the drug. If you have acute disease, you may need medication for only a few weeks. Chronic bacterial prostatitis, on the other hand, is often more resistant to antibiotics, making the drugs less effective. It takes longer to cure the infection, and sometimes it can't be cured. In addition, you may have a relapse as soon as the drug is withdrawn. If this happens, you may need to take a low-dose antibiotic daily for an indefinite period to keep the infection under control.

Even though nonbacterial prostatitis isn't caused by an infection, some doctors will prescribe an antibiotic for a few weeks to see if it helps improve symptoms. If the drug doesn't help, your doctor will recommend that you stop taking it. If your symptoms do improve, your doctor may suggest continuing the medication for a few more weeks. Some people with nonbacterial prostatitis find a continuous, low dose of an antibiotic helps to prevent symptoms, or reduce their severity. How or why the medication helps is unknown.

Alpha-blockers. If you're having difficulty urinating, perhaps due to an obstruction in your urinary tract, your doctor may prescribe an alpha-blocker. Alpha-blockers help relax the prostate and bladder neck, improving urine flow. Because you're able to eliminate more urine, they may reduce the number of times you need to go to the bathroom at night.

Pain relievers. An over-the-counter pain reliever, such as aspirin, a nonsteroidal anti-inflammatory drug (NSAID), or acetaminophen can help relieve pain and discomfort. However, discuss with your doctor how much of the drug to take to avoid side effects.

Physical therapy

Stretching and relaxing the lower pelvic muscles helps to relieve symptoms in some men. A physical therapist can provide guidance on which exercises are beneficial and how to perform them. Heat, in the form of diathermy, may be included in your treatment sessions. This process uses electrical currents to heat tissues in the muscles, making them more limber and easier to relax. After working with a physical therapist, you continue to do the exercises on your own at home.

Your therapist also may try other relaxation techniques, such as biofeedback. Biofeedback uses technology to teach you how to control certain body responses, including relaxing your muscles. During a biofeedback session, a trained therapist applies electrodes and other sensors to skin located on various parts of your body. The electrodes are attached to a monitor that gives you feedback on bodily functions, including muscle tension. Once the electrodes are in place, the therapist uses relaxation techniques to calm you, reducing muscle tension. You then learn how to produce these changes yourself.

Doctors aren't sure why physical therapy works for prostatitis. They speculate that among some men, tight or irritated muscles may be a contributing factor to their condition.

Sitz baths
Many men find these baths can relieve their pain and relax the pelvic and lower abdominal muscles. From the German word sitzen, meaning "to sit," this type of bath simply involves sitting and soaking the lower half of your body in warm water.

Common but unproven practices

Because chronic prostatitis is both difficult to understand and to treat, over the years men have experimented with various lifestyle changes to control their symptoms. Some more common practices include:

- Drinking plenty of water
- Limiting alcohol, caffeine and highly spiced foods
- Going to the bathroom at regular intervals
- Having frequent sexual intercourse

While these practices don't cause any harm, there's no scientific evidence to prove they're beneficial. Studies have yet to show that changes in dietary, bathroom or sexual habits can cure prostatitis or relieve your symptoms.

This doesn't mean, however, that if you find such practices helpful you should discontinue them. For reasons that are unclear, some men find simple things, such as avoiding long periods of sitting or certain foods or beverages, seem to improve their condition.

For many men with prostatitis, living with the disease often boils down to limiting those things that seem to make the condition worse and doing others that seem to improve it, without knowing why or how the changes help.

Getting relief from chronic prostatitis can be a long process that may take months. The condition also can recur for no apparent reason.

When your condition is first diagnosed, your doctor may recommend taking sitz baths two or three times a day for 30 minutes each time. For acute prostatitis, keep the water temperature below 99 F. If you have chronic disease, temperatures up to 115 F are fine.

Prostate massage

Massaging the prostate can often help to relieve congestion in the gland due to an infection and to unplug tiny ducts blocked by bacteria. In addition, massage may improve the effectiveness of antibiotics by making it easier for the drugs to penetrate more deeply into infected tissues.

When it's really not prostatitis

Sometimes men who see a doctor for what appears to be prostatitis don't have prostatitis but another condition called prostatodynia (PROS-tuh-toe-DIN-ee-uh). Men with this condition often refer to their symptoms as pain "down there," meaning anywhere in the genital area. The symptoms typically mimic those of chronic nonbacterial prostatitis. The difference between the two conditions is that with prostatodynia, urine and prostate fluid samples don't indicate any evidence of infection or inflammation. Bacteria or white blood cells aren't detectable in the samples.

Rather than being a problem with your prostate gland, prostatodynia may instead stem from your pelvic floor muscles. When you're under stress, you may not completely relax those muscles supporting your bladder and urethra, causing difficulties when you urinate. This theory could explain why most men who have prostatodynia tend to have type A personalities — hard-driven, tense, stressed. Prostatodynia also seems to occur more frequently among marathon runners, bicyclists, triathletes, weight lifters and truck drivers.

Treatment for prostatodynia is similar in many ways to treatment for nonbacterial prostatitis. Physical therapy to help relax your pelvic floor muscles is generally the first step. Your doctor may also recommend stress management courses to help you learn to prevent and better cope with stress.

An alpha-blocker to relax muscles in your prostate and bladder neck may be helpful. Some men remain on the drug indefinitely, because their symptoms return as soon as it's withdrawn. You might also try sitz baths to see if they improve your symptoms.

Answers to your questions

Does prostatitis increase my risk of cancer?
There's no evidence that having acute or chronic prostatitis puts you at greater risk of prostate cancer. Prostatitis does, however, increase the level of prostate-specific antigen in your blood. If your PSA level is elevated and you have prostatitis, it's advisable to redo the test after you've been treated with antibiotics. If you have chronic prostatitis, ask your doctor about the value of having a free-PSA test (see page 20).

Can I pass on a prostate infection to my partner during intercourse?
Prostatitis can result from a sexually transmitted disease, but prostatitis itself isn't contagious. Prostatitis can't be passed on through sexual intercourse, so your partner doesn't have to worry about "catching" the infection.

Can prostatitis make me infertile?
It may. The disease can interfere with the development of semen, making it difficult for the fluid to ejaculate properly during intercourse. Because semen carries sperm, this may lower your fertility rate. A few studies also indicate poor sperm quality in some men with prostatitis.

Is surgery ever used to treat the disease?
Generally, doctors prefer nonsurgical procedures. But if the disease has drastically affected your fertility or antibiotics aren't able to improve your symptoms, your doctor might recommend surgery. A surgeon may try to open blocked ducts in the gland to relieve

congestion and help semen flow more freely. Surgery is not recommended for nonbacterial disease.

Can the herb saw palmetto help relieve my symptoms?
Studies show that saw palmetto may be an effective treatment for noncancerous enlargement of the prostate gland (benign prostatic hyperplasia). However, there's no evidence that this popular herb relieves infection or inflammation associated with prostatitis. Saw palmetto is discussed later in this book on page 154.

Chapter 4

Understanding Benign Prostatic Hyperplasia (BPH)

A t birth, your prostate gland is about the size of a pea. It grows slightly during childhood and then at puberty undergoes a rapid growth spurt. By the time you reach age 25, your prostate is fully developed.

Most men, however, experience a second period of prostate growth. When they reach their mid-40s, cells in the central portion of the gland — where the prostate surrounds the urethra — begin to reproduce more rapidly than normal. As tissues in the area enlarge, they often press on the urethra and obstruct urine flow (see illustration). Benign prostatic hyperplasia is the medical term for this condition. It's more commonly called BPH.

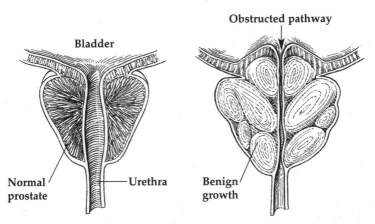

The urethra, the tube that drains the bladder, is surrounded by the prostate gland. Benign prostatic hyperplasia results when tissues in the center portion of the prostate enlarge and press on the urethra, affecting normal urine flow.

A common fact of life

The chances that BPH will develop grow right along with your age. BPH affects about half of men in their 60s and close to 80 percent of men in their 80s.

The causes of prostate enlargement are unclear. Researchers believe that as your prostate ages, it becomes more susceptible to the effects of male hormones, including testosterone. These hormones make certain prostate tissues grow.

Other factors likely play a role. A family history of BPH can increase your odds for the disease, pointing to a possible genetic link. BPH is more common in American and European men than in men of Asian descent. This suggests a possible lifestyle component. For unknown reasons, married men are more likely to get BPH than single men.

Fortunately, the condition varies in severity and doesn't always pose a problem. Only about half of men with BPH experience symptoms that become noticeable or annoying enough for them to seek medical treatment. These symptoms may include:

- A weak urine stream
- Difficulty starting urinating
- Stopping and starting again while urinating
- Dribbling at the end of urination
- Frequent or urgent need to urinate
- Increased urination at night (nocturia)
- Not being able to empty the bladder

Only if it prevents you from emptying your bladder can BPH become a serious health threat. A bladder that's continually full can result in recurrent bladder infection and kidney damage.

In about half of men with BPH, symptoms stay the same or improve. Among the other half, they gradually worsen.

Seeing a doctor

If you're experiencing urinary problems, make an appointment to see your doctor, or mention your symptoms at an upcoming visit.

Your doctor can determine whether you have BPH and your symptoms warrant treatment. If you don't find your symptoms annoying and they don't pose a health threat, treatment may not be necessary. That doesn't mean, however, that it's all right to let urinary symptoms go unchecked. Instead of BPH, your symptoms could be early warnings of a more serious condition, including a bladder stone, a bladder infection, side effects of medication, heart failure, diabetes, a neurologic problem, prostatitis or prostate cancer.

Your doctor will likely begin by asking you questions about your symptoms, when they developed, and how often they occur. He or she also will want to know about other health problems you may have, medications you may be taking, and whether there's a history of prostate problems in your family. In addition, your checkup may include:

- A digital rectal exam to see whether your prostate is enlarged and to help rule out prostate cancer
- A urine test to rule out an infection or condition that can produce similar symptoms
- A PSA blood test to help rule out prostate cancer

Getting a diagnosis

If the results of the previous tests suggest BPH, your doctor may want to perform some additional exams. They can help confirm the diagnosis of BPH and determine its severity.

AUA symptom index
This is a short questionnaire developed by the American Urological Association. It asks you about specific urinary symptoms associated with BPH and how often they occur (see "How you do you rate?" on the following page).

Urinary flow test
This test measures the strength and amount of your urine flow. A flow rate of more than 15 milliliters per second (mL/sec) is normal or signifies only mild disease. A rate of 10 to 15 mL/sec is often

How do you rate?

The American Urological Association has devised this worksheet to help doctors evaluate BPH severity.

Questions	Not at all	Less than 1 time in 5	Less than half the time	About half the time	More than half the time	Almost always	Score
Over the past month, how often have you had a sensation of not emptying your bladder completely after you finished urinating?	0	1	2	3	4	5	_____
Over the past month, how often have you had to urinate again less than 2 hours after you had finished urinating?	0	1	2	3	4	5	_____
Over the past month, how often have you found you stopped and started again several times when you urinated?	0	1	2	3	4	5	_____
Over the past month, how often have you found it is difficult to postpone urination?	0	1	2	3	4	5	_____
Over the past month, how often have you had a weak urinary stream?	0	1	2	3	4	5	_____
Over the past month, how often have you had to push or strain to begin urination?	0	1	2	3	4	5	_____
	None	1 Time	2 Times	3 Times	4 Times	5 or more times	
Over the past month, how many times did you most typically get up to urinate from the time you went to bed at night until you got up in the morning?	0	1	2	3	4	5	_____

Total Score _____

Scoring Key

Mild symptoms: 0 to 7 total points
Moderate symptoms: 8 to 19 total points
Severe symptoms: 20 to 35 total points

associated with moderate symptoms. Anything less than 10 mL/sec usually indicates severe BPH.

By charting the results of this test, your doctor can determine if your urinary flow patterns are worsening over time, and at what speed. Keep in mind, however, that your flow rate normally decreases as you age. Restricted urine flow also can be a sign of other problems, such as weak bladder muscle.

Post-void residual volume test

This test measures whether you can empty your bladder. The test is done one of two ways: by inserting a small catheter into your urethra and up into your bladder or by using ultrasound imaging to see inside your bladder.

The ultrasound method is more common but less accurate. Because the results of this test can vary, you may need to have it done more than once to get an accurate reading.

Ultrasound

Ultrasound imaging also is used to estimate the size of your prostate gland. In addition, it can detect problems such as a kidney obstruction, stones in your kidneys or prostate, or a tumor.

Urodynamic studies

If your doctor suspects that your symptoms may be related to a bladder problem rather than BPH, he or she may recommend a series of tests to measure bladder pressure and function.

These tests are done by threading a small catheter through the urethra and into the bladder. Bladder pressure is measured during urination. Water also is injected into your bladder to measure internal bladder pressure and to determine how effectively your bladder contracts.

Cystoscopy

This procedure involves use of a thin tube containing a lens with a light system (cystoscope) that's inserted into the urethra. It allows your doctor to see inside the urethra, bladder and prostate. The procedure can detect problems including enlargement of the prostate, obstruction of the urethra or bladder neck, an anatomic abnormality or the development of stones in your bladder.

Intravenous pyelogram

An intravenous pyelogram (PIE-uh-low-gram) is an X-ray image of the urinary tract used to help detect an obstruction or abnormality. Dye is injected into a vein and an X-ray taken of your kidneys, bladder and the tubes that attach your kidneys to your bladder (ureters). The dye makes it possible to identify a blockage. Because of newer imaging techniques and risk of an allergic reaction to the dye, this procedure is used less often today.

Answers to your questions

Are the tests used to diagnose BPH painful?
Most aren't painful. But you may experience mild discomfort. Sometimes a local anesthetic is used to minimize the discomfort.

Do men with larger prostates generally have more severe symptoms?
No. This is a common misconception. You can have a very large prostate gland with few or no symptoms, or a small gland with severe symptoms. That's because BPH results from growth in the center portion of the prostate, not the outside. While it may squeeze inside tissues, the growth doesn't always affect the overall dimensions of the gland.

Does BPH increase my odds of having cancer?
There's no evidence that BPH increases your risk of prostate cancer. The two conditions appear to develop independently of each other.

Chapter 5

Treating Benign Prostatic Hyperplasia

D
o you avoid social events so you won't have to worry about long lines to the bathroom? Are you tired in the morning from getting up during the night to go to the bathroom? Are you no longer wearing dark-colored pants for fear of noticeable dribbling? These are common ways benign prostatic hyperplasia (BPH) can interfere with your life.

Many men would rather put up with the inconveniences of BPH than treat it. But if your symptoms have reached the point where they're affecting your quality of life, it may be time to see a doctor. Treatment for BPH comes in various forms.

Watchful waiting

If your symptoms are mild and you're not bothered by them, you and your doctor may decide that "watchful waiting" is appropriate. Your doctor will periodically evaluate your condition to see if it improves, stays the same or worsens.

The advantage of watchful waiting is you don't have to undergo any invasive treatment. Your treatment usually doesn't cost you anything beyond the usual fees for your physical examination and perhaps some tests. The risk you take is that your condition could worsen drastically or other problems may develop, such as an infection. But this is uncommon.

While you wait

Some simple lifestyle changes can often help control symptoms of BPH and prevent your condition from worsening.

Limit beverages. Stop drinking water and other beverages after 7 p.m. to reduce your need to go to the bathroom at night.

Empty your bladder. Try to urinate all that you can each time you go to the bathroom.

Limit alcohol. It increases urine production and may cause congestion in the prostate gland.

Be careful with over-the-counter decongestants. They can cause the band of muscle that controls urine flow from your urethra (urethral sphincter) to tighten, making urination more difficult.

Keep active. Inactivity causes you to retain urine. A recent study shows that even a small amount of exercise can reduce urinary problems caused by BPH.

Stay warm. Cold weather can lead to urine retention.

Medication

Pharmaceutical companies have invested hundreds of millions of dollars to develop drugs for prostate enlargement. As a result, medication is now the most common method for controlling moderate symptoms of BPH. Medication is also an option for men with mild BPH who find their symptoms annoying or men who don't care for watchful waiting.

There are two types of medications for BPH:

Alpha-blockers

These drugs were originally developed to treat high blood pressure, but they're also beneficial for other conditions, including BPH. They relax your muscles, including your pelvic muscles, making it easier to urinate. The Food and Drug Administration has approved three types of alpha-blockers for BPH:

- Terazosin (Hytrin)
- Doxazosin (Cardura)
- Tamsulosin (Flomax)

Alpha-blockers are effective in about 75 percent of men who take them. The drugs also work quickly. Within just 1 or 2 days, most men notice an increase in urinary flow and a decrease in how often they need to urinate.

Doctors still are uncertain about the long-term benefits and risks of alpha-blockers. However, the drugs appear to be safe. Side effects can include headaches or feeling dizzy, light-headed or tired. For this reason, it's best to take the medication before bedtime. Some men also report trouble getting an erection (impotence), and feeling faint when standing too quickly, due to low blood pressure (hypotension). To reduce your risk of these side effects, your doctor may start you out with a low dose of medication and gradually increase the dosage.

Tamsulosin, the newest of the three drugs, may cause less dizziness. You also don't need to gradually increase its dosage. As result, its benefits tend to be more noticeable and occur more quickly. Abnormal ejaculation can occur in men who take tamsulosin. However, adjusting the dosage may remedy the problem.

Finasteride

Finasteride (Proscar) relieves BPH symptoms in a totally different manner. Instead of relaxing your pelvic muscles, it shrinks your prostate gland. For some men with large prostates, the drug may produce a noticeable improvement in symptoms. It's generally not effective, though, if you have a moderately enlarged or normal-sized prostate.

Finasteride takes a long time to work. You may notice some improvement in urinary flow after 3 months, but it generally takes up to a year for complete results. A small percentage of men who take finasteride experience impotence, decreased libido, and reduced semen release during ejaculation. But in most men it produces only slight side effects. Long-term effects of the medication are unknown.

Finasteride has two other drawbacks. It's more expensive than alpha-blockers, and it lowers your prostate-specific antigen (PSA) level. This can interfere with the effectiveness of the PSA screening test for prostate cancer.

Surgery

At one time, surgery was the most common treatment for BPH. But because of increased use of medications and the development of other less invasive therapies, surgery is on the decline. Today, it's used mainly for more severe symptoms or if you have complicating factors, such as:

- Frequent urinary tract infections
- Kidney damage from urinary retention
- Bleeding through the urethra
- Stones in the bladder

Surgery is the most effective of all therapies for relieving symptoms of BPH. It's the "gold standard" by which all other treatments are judged. However, it's also the most likely to produce side effects. Fortunately, most men experience few problems. Among people with certain health conditions, such as uncontrolled diabetes, cirrhosis of the liver, a major psychiatric disorder, or serious lung, kidney or heart conditions, surgery isn't usually recommended.

There are three types of surgery for BPH:

TURP

Transurethral resection of the prostate (TURP) is the most common. During the procedure, you're placed under general anesthesia or anesthetized from the waist down with a spinal block. A surgeon threads a narrow instrument (resectoscope) into the urethra and uses small cutting tools to scrape away excess prostate tissue (see illustration). You can expect to stay in the hospital for 1 to 3 days following surgery. During recovery you'll have a urinary catheter for a few days.

TURP is effective and relieves symptoms quickly. Most men experience a stronger urine flow within a few days. You can expect some blood or small blood clots to appear in your urine afterward. Before you leave the hospital you should be able to urinate on your own. At first you may feel some pain or a sense of urgency when urine passes over the surgical area. This discomfort should gradually improve.

In a few cases, TURP can cause impotence and loss of bladder control. These conditions are generally only temporary. Pelvic floor muscle exercises (Kegel exercises) will often help restore bladder control (see page 102). Normal sexual function often returns within a few weeks to months. However, it can take up to a year for full recovery.

Another more common side effect of surgery is retrograde ejaculation. In this condition, semen flows backward into your bladder during orgasm instead of out through the penis, causing infertility. TURP also may produce scarring and narrowing in the urethra. This often can be remedied by a simple stretching procedure done on an outpatient basis.

Up to 10 percent of men who have TURP need surgery again within 10 years, because the prostate tissue grows back.

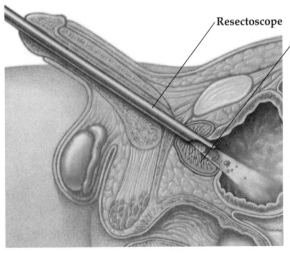

Resectoscope   BPH

Transurethral resection of the prostate (TURP) is the most common surgery for BPH. A thin instrument (resectoscope) is threaded through the urethra to where it's surrounded by the prostate. Tiny cutting tools on the resectoscope scrape away excess prostate tissue, improving urine flow.

TUIP

Transurethral incision of the prostate (TUIP) is an option if you have a moderately enlarged or small prostate gland. It's also an option for men who aren't good candidates for more invasive surgery for health reasons or because they don't want to risk sterility from retrograde ejaculation.

Like TURP, TUIP involves special instruments that are inserted through the urethra. But instead of removing prostate tissue, the surgeon makes one or two small cuts in the prostate gland. The cuts help enlarge the opening of the urethra, making it easier to urinate.

The procedure produces less risk of complications than other kinds of surgery and it doesn't require an overnight hospital stay. However, it's less effective and it often needs to be repeated. Some men experience only a small improvement in urinary flow.

Open prostatectomy

This type of surgery is generally performed only if you have an excessively large prostate, you have bladder damage, or you have other complicating factors, such as stones in your bladder. It's called "open" because the surgeon makes an incision in your lower abdomen to reach the prostate, rather than going up through the urethra.

Open prostatectomy is the most effective therapy for relieving BPH. However, it also poses the greatest risk of side effects. Complications of the procedure are similar to those of TURP, and their effects may be more severe. The procedure usually requires a hospital stay of 5 to 10 days.

The most common type of open prostatectomy is radical prostatectomy to remove a cancerous prostate. It involves removing the entire prostate gland. During a partial prostatectomy for the treatment of BPH, only the inner portion of the gland is removed, leaving the outer portion intact.

Recovering from surgery

Depending on the type of surgery you have, it may take a couple of weeks to a few months for a full recovery. During this time, it's often best to avoid activities that involve lifting, jarring to your pelvic area, such as from operating heavy equipment or riding a bicycle, and straining of your lower abdominal muscles, such as during a bowel movement.

To prevent constipation, eat plenty of high-fiber foods, such as fruits, vegetables and grains. Fiber softens stool and makes it easier to pass. Drinking eight glasses of water daily also helps cleanse your urinary tract and promote healing.

Heat therapy (thermotherapy)

These are less invasive treatments that use heat energy to destroy excessive prostate tissue. Thermotherapy fills the gap between medication and invasive surgery. It's more effective than medication for moderate to severe symptoms, and it doesn't produce as many side effects as surgery.

There are several types of thermotherapy:

Microwave therapy

Transurethral microwave therapy (TUMT) uses computer-controlled heat in the form of microwave energy to safely destroy the inner portion of the enlarged gland.

During the procedure, a machine emits microwave energy through a urinary catheter. The catheter includes a tiny internal microwave antenna to deliver a dose of microwave energy that heats the enlarged cells and destroys them. Cool water circulates around the tip and sides of the antenna during the procedure to protect the urethra from the heat.

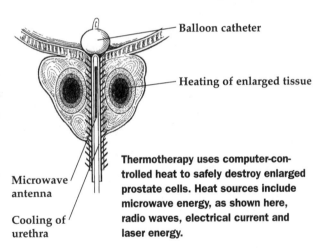

Thermotherapy uses computer-controlled heat to safely destroy enlarged prostate cells. Heat sources include microwave energy, as shown here, radio waves, electrical current and laser energy.

A local anesthetic helps control pain. You may feel some heat in the prostate and bladder area. You also may have a strong desire to urinate and may experience bladder spasms. These responses are usually well tolerated and disappear after the treatment is finished. You can go home when you're urinating satisfactorily — usually the same day of your treatment. About 30 percent of men need to wear a urinary catheter for a few days.

Unlike TURP, it may take several weeks before you begin to see a noticeable improvement in your symptoms. The long-term effectiveness of the procedure is also uncertain. One study found that 60 percent to 70 percent of men respond well to TUMT initially, but only about 25 percent of the men were satisfied with the results 4 years later. Those who seem to respond best over time are men whose initial symptoms are mild.

It's normal to have urgency, frequent urination and small amounts of blood in your urine during recovery. You also may experience a change in the amount of semen you ejaculate. However, unlike more invasive surgery, TUMT generally doesn't produce impotence, incontinence or retrograde ejaculation.

The procedure isn't recommended if you have a pacemaker or any metal implants.

Radiofrequency therapy

Transurethral needle ablation (TUNA) works by sending radio waves through needles that are inserted into the prostate gland, heating and destroying the tissue. As in TUMT, a special catheter is inserted through your urethra. The needles are inserted into the prostate by maneuvering the catheter.

TUNA typically is less effective than traditional surgery in reducing symptoms and improving urine flow. Its long-term effectiveness also isn't known. Another drawback of the procedure is that it doesn't work as well in men with large prostates.

The procedure, however, doesn't produce incontinence or impotence. Side effects may include urine retention, blood in your urine, painful urination, and a small risk of retrograde ejaculation.

Heating better than freezing

Another approach to destroying prostate tissue is freezing the tissue, rather than heating it. During a procedure called cryosurgery, extremely cold liquid nitrogen is injected into the prostate gland by way of five tiny probes.

Cryosurgery was once a fairly popular treatment option, but its use and appeal have diminished as studies show that it isn't as effective as surgery or thermotherapy for improving urine flow.

Electrovaporization

Transurethral electrovaporization of the prostate (TVP) is a modification of the TURP procedure that provides nearly bloodless removal of prostate tissue, along with a shorter hospital stay and less catheterization time.

It involves a special metal instrument that emits a high-frequency electrical current to cut and vaporize excess tissue, while sealing off the tissue to prevent bleeding.

TVP may be as effective as TURP, without the high cost and with fewer complications. Because this type of surgery is technically simpler and causes so little bleeding, it's useful for men at higher risk of complications, including those taking blood-thinning medication.

As with other less invasive treatments, its long-term benefits aren't yet known.

Laser therapy

Laser therapy is performed similarly to other thermotherapies, but it uses a laser instead of microwave energy, radio waves or electrical current to produce heat. It generally doesn't cause impotence or prolonged incontinence. However, some laser procedures require lengthy use of a catheter.

TUEP. Transurethral evaporation of the prostate (TUEP) is similar to electrovaporization. The difference is that your doctor uses laser energy to destroy prostate tissue instead of electrical current. The procedure is generally safe and causes limited bleeding. It's often effective, with noticeable improvement in urine flow soon after the procedure.

VLAP. Visual laser ablation of the prostate (VLAP) involves applying enough laser energy to dry up and destroy excess prostate cells, which you eventually eliminate over several weeks to months. One major drawback lessens its appeal: Because of swelling and prolonged sloughing off of the dead tissue, you're likely to retain urine for several days and will need to wear a catheter. You may also experience a burning sensation for days to weeks during urination.

Interstitial laser therapy. This particular procedure directs laser energy inside the benign tumors rather than at the urethral surface.

> **Building a better laser**
>
> One of the biggest drawbacks to laser therapy is the need for a catheter for a prolonged period following treatment. New types of lasers are helping resolve this problem.
>
> The newer lasers work two ways: They both cut out and vaporize excess prostate tissue. This allows immediate removal of obstructive tissue, so you only need a catheter for 24 hours at most. Two such lasers being evaluated include the KTP laser and the Holmium: YAG laser. Mayo Clinic urologists have pioneered the use of the KTP laser with continued success.
>
> The goal is to combine the advantages of laser therapy — safety and limited bleeding — with immediate improvement in urinary flow that comes with more invasive surgery.

It safely and moderately increases the urinary flow rate, and reduces the volume of the prostate. It also seems to work well among men with large prostates.

Because of substantial tissue inflammation after treatment, you may need to use a catheter for up to 3 weeks. Uncomplicated urinary tract infections also are common. Interstitital laser therapy doesn't cause any blood loss and is a good option if you can't have surgery.

Nonsurgical procedures

For men who are unwilling or unable to take medication or who are reluctant or unable to have surgery, these options also exist:

Balloon dilation

With the use of a catheter, your doctor positions a tiny deflated balloon in the part of your urethra that lies within your prostate gland. The balloon is then inflated to stretch the urethra and compress prostate tissue. However, because the improvement lasts only a short time, use of this procedure has declined.

Prostatic stents

A tiny metal coil is inserted into your urethra to widen the urethra and keep it open. Tissue grows over the stent to hold it in place.

One advantage of the procedure is that it lasts only 10 to 15 minutes. It also produces little or no bleeding and doesn't require a catheter. In early trials, though, nearly one-third of the men with stents had them removed because of poor placement or complications. Some men found that the stents didn't improve their symptoms. Others experienced irritation when urinating or had frequent urinary tract infections.

These complications, along with the high cost and potential difficulties in removing the stents, have reduced their popularity.

A BPH shot?

Because BPH is such a common problem, new and better therapies to treat the condition are constantly being explored. Transurethral enzyme injection (TUEI) is one therapy that may play a role in future treatment. By way of a catheter, a combination of enzymes is injected into your prostate to dissolve the extra tissue. Studies in animals suggest that the procedure is effective, safe, and worthy of testing in humans. Mayo Clinic is among those institutions experimenting with the drug combination.

Researchers also are experimenting with purified alcohol that's injected into the benign tumors. In an effort to dilute the alcohol, prostate cells absorb additional water. However, the cells take in so much water that they explode and die.

Weighing your options

With so many options to choose from, deciding on the best way to treat BPH can be difficult. There isn't really one therapy that stands out above the rest. Each treatment may improve your symptoms, but in different ways. Each also has its advantages and disadvantages. The question becomes which one will best meet your needs with the fewest side effects. As you and your doctor plan your treatment strategy, consider these important factors:

Severity of your symptoms

If your symptoms don't bother you and your condition isn't causing any other problems, you can probably wait to see if your symptoms improve or worsen. On the other hand, if you have severe symptoms, organ damage or complicating factors, such as frequent urinary infections, bleeding or bladder stones, you may need surgery.

Treatment for anything between these two choices depends on your personal preference. Will you settle for a small improvement in symptoms, or are you hoping for something more noticeable? Do you want immediate relief or can you wait? Are you willing to take medication daily? Will you tolerate some side effects?

Size of your gland

Some treatments are best suited for large prostates (30 to 40 grams and larger). Others are more effective for smaller to moderately sized prostates. Therapies best suited for large prostates include:
- Finasteride (Proscar)
- Transurethral resection of the prostate (TURP)
- Open prostatectomy
- Transurethral microwave therapy (TUMT)
- Laser therapy

Treatments more appropriate for small to moderately sized prostates include:
- Alpha-blockers
- Transurethral incision of the prostate (TUIP)
- Transurethral needle ablation (TUNA)
- Transurethral electrovaporization of the prostate (TVP)
- Laser therapy

Your age

The best treatment for a man in his 50s may not be the best for a man in his 80s. If you're younger, you may want a treatment that provides long-term benefits. If you're older, immediate benefits may be more important than long-term effects. In addition, younger men often recover more quickly from surgery and other invasive procedures than men in their 70s or 80s.

Your health

If you have other health conditions, you may not be a good candidate for surgery or recover as quickly. Surgery generally isn't recommended if you have:

- Uncontrolled diabetes
- Cirrhosis of the liver
- Serious lung, kidney or heart disease
- A major psychiatric disorder

Some people aren't good candidates for medication because of intolerance to a specific drug or certain kinds of medication.

Your fertility

If you want to father children, you'll want to avoid therapies that could cause infertility. TURP, TUIP, open prostatectomy and laser therapy can lead to retrograde ejaculation, in which semen backs up into your bladder instead of ejaculating from your penis. Your risk of retrograde ejaculation after surgery is between 30 percent and 90 percent. Unlike impotence, which may only be temporary, retrograde ejaculation is usually permanent.

In rare cases, TUNA, interstitial laser therapy and alpha-blockers can cause retrograde ejaculation.

Your sexuality

Surgery can damage nerves or blood vessels located next to the prostate gland, causing impotence. Your odds of experiencing impotence following TURP are about 10 percent. Often, however, normal sexual function returns after a few months.

Impotence — even for a short time — is a concern for many men. Discuss this issue with your doctor before surgery.

Benefits vs. risks

Do the benefits of the procedure you're considering outweigh the risks? (See "A brief comparison" on page 55.)

TURP is the most effective treatment for BPH, in large part because it has been used for years and doctors know its long-term effects. But it also poses some risks. In addition to impotence and retrograde ejaculation, it causes urinary tract infections in about 16 percent of men and incontinence in about 1 percent. Open prostatectomy has even greater benefits and risks, but because it's more invasive it's less commonly used.

Less invasive thermotherapies appear to be effective, and they generally produce fewer side effects. But because these therapies are newer, their long-term benefits still aren't fully known.

As for medication, alpha-blockers appear to offer long-term benefits. However, the drugs can cause side effects in some men.

Expertise of your doctor

You want to select a therapy in which your doctor has considerable knowledge. Generally, the more experience your doctor has with the therapy, the less risk of side effects and the greater your odds for noticeable improvement.

Recovery time

Recovery varies with the treatment. If you choose medication, you don't have to worry about being laid up or missing work.

Thermotherapy is often performed on an outpatient basis. However, depending on the procedure, your doctor, and how quickly you're able to urinate on your own, you may need to stay in the hospital overnight. Thermotherapy ordinarily requires only a few days' recovery time. An exception is laser therapy. Some older laser procedures require that you wear a catheter for up to 3 weeks. Newer techniques often require use of a catheter for only 24 hours.

Surgery for BPH requires a hospital stay. Plan for a 5- to 10-day stay if you have open prostatectomy. TURP may mean a stay of 3 to 5 days, and TUIP 1 to 3 days in the hospital. In some cases, TUIP is done on an outpatient basis.

If you have surgery, you may need to take up to a month off from work. For up to 2 months, you'll also need to avoid heavy lifting, jarring to your lower pelvic area, or straining of your lower abdominal muscles.

A brief comparison

Treatment	Advantages	Disadvantages
Watchful waiting	Causes no side effects or complications.	Symptoms could become more severe.
Alpha-blockers	Help 3 out of 4 men. Work quickly.	Can cause mild flulike symptoms. Long-term effects not fully known.
Finasteride	Causes few side effects.	Most effective in larger prostates. Works slowly. Long-term effects unknown.
Transurethral resection of the prostate (TURP)	Most common form of surgery. Effective and provides immediate results.	Requires 1-3 day hospital stay. Small risk of impotence and incontinence. Causes retrograde ejaculation.
Transurethral incision of the prostate (TUIP)	An outpatient procedure. Fewer side effects. Doesn't cause retrograde ejaculation.	Not as effective as TURP. Less effective in men with large prostates.
Open prostatectomy	Most effective therapy.	Greatest risk of side effects. Lengthy hospital stay.
Microwave therapy	Generally effective. Fewer side effects than TURP. An outpatient procedure.	Results can take several weeks. Long-term effects uncertain.
Radiofrequency therapy	Generally effective. Causes few side effects. An outpatient procedure.	Less effective in larger prostates. Results take time. Long-term effects unknown.
Electrovaporization	Similar in effectiveness to TURP. Few side effects. Doesn't cause blood loss.	Requires 1-2 day hospital stay. Long-term effects unknown.
Laser therapy	As effective as TURP. Newer lasers cause minimal side effects. Outpatient procedure.	Some older forms of treatment can require lengthy use of a catheter.
Balloon dilation	Doesn't require surgery. No side effects.	Effects last only a short time.
Stents	Doesn't require surgery. Quick procedure.	Often not effective. Can cause bothersome side effects.

Answers to your questions

Can treatment for BPH reduce my risk of getting cancer?
No. BPH treatments don't reduce the risk of prostate cancer, with
the exception of complete prostate removal. Even if you're being
treated for BPH, you still need to continue regular prostate exams
to screen for cancer. Surgery for BPH, however, can identify cancer
in its early stages. Unsuspected cancer is found during surgery in
about 15 percent of men.

Is Proscar the same drug used for hair growth?
Yes. Proscar (finasteride) is the same as Propecia. The only differ-
ence is the dose. Proscar comes in a 5 milligram (mg) tablet,
Propecia in a 1 mg tablet.

If the first option I choose doesn't work, can I try another?
Absolutely. Conservative options, such as medication, are often the
first choice of many men and their doctors. If they don't produce
satisfactory results, then you can move on to an invasive procedure.

Should I get a second opinion before deciding on a treatment?
Not necessarily. It depends on the confidence you have in your
doctor and the therapeutic option that you choose. If you select a
more conservative therapy such as medication or thermotherapy,
your doctor has adequate experience with the therapy, and you feel
comfortable with the decision, a second opinion may not be necessary. If you don't feel comfortable with your doctor's recommendation, then it might be a good idea to consult another doctor.

Is it OK to take part in an experimental study?
Yes. Experimental studies can give you the opportunity to receive
the benefits of new, innovative treatments. But before enrolling in a
study, make sure you fully understand the possible side effects of
the procedure as well as its potential benefits.

Part 3

Prostate Cancer

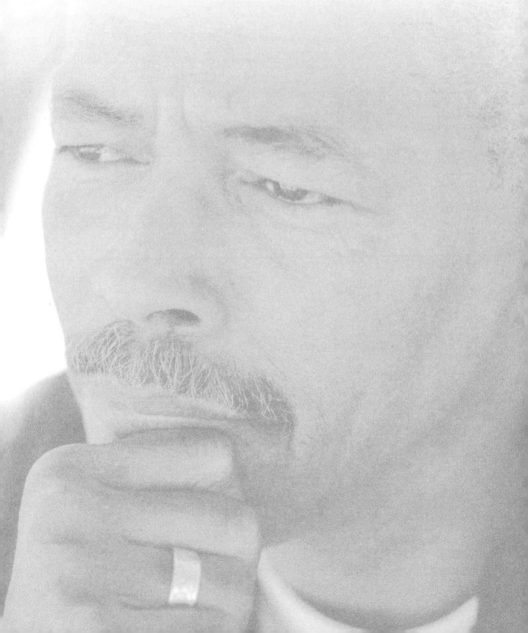

Chapter 6

Learning You Have Cancer

Prostate cancer is the most common cancer in American men. (Basal and squamous cell skin cancers are actually diagnosed more often, but these cancers aren't life-threatening.) It's estimated that by age 50, up to 1 in 4 men have some cancerous cells in the prostate gland. By age 80, the ratio increases to 1 in 2. As you age, your risk of prostate cancer increases. The average age at diagnosis of prostate cancer is 72.

Prostate cancer also is the second leading cause of cancer deaths in American men — not because it's so deadly, but because it's so common. Unlike other cancers, you're more likely to die *with* prostate cancer than you are *of* it. On average, an American man has about a 30 percent risk of having prostate cancer, but only about a 3 percent risk of dying of the disease.

What exactly is cancer?

Cancer, simply put, is a group of abnormal cells that grow more rapidly than normal cells and refuse to die. Your body continuously produces new cells that live only a short time before being replaced by fresh cells. Skin cells, for example, live just a few weeks. But microscopic cancer cells grow into small nodules or pea-size collections that continue to grow, becoming more densely packed and hard.

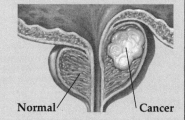

Normal   Cancer

Cancer Facts and Figures

Cancer Cases by Site and Sex

MALE	FEMALE
Prostate 179,300	Breast 175,000
Lung & bronchus 94,000	Lung & bronchus 77,600
Colon & rectum 62,400	Colon & rectum 67,000
Urinary bladder 39,100	Uterine corpus 37,400
Non-Hodgkin's lymphoma 32,600	Ovary 25,200
Melanoma of the skin 25,800	Non-Hodgkin's lymphoma 24,200
Oral cavity 20,000	Melanoma of the skin 18,400
Kidney 17,800	Urinary bladder 15,100
Leukemia 16,800	Pancreas 14,600
Pancreas 14,000	Thyroid 13,500
All sites 623,800	All sites 598,000

Cancer Deaths by Site and Sex

MALE	FEMALE
Lung & bronchus 90,900	Lung & bronchus 68,000
Prostate 37,000	Breast 43,300
Colon & rectum 27,800	Colon & rectum 28,800
Pancreas 13,900	Pancreas 14,700
Non-Hodgkin's lymphoma 13,400	Ovary 14,500
Leukemia 12,400	Non-Hodgkin's lymphoma 12,300
Esophagus 9,400	Leukemia 9,700
Liver 8,400	Uterine corpus 6,400
Urinary bladder 8,100	Brain 5,900
Stomach 7,900	Stomach 5,600
All sites 291,100	All sites 272,000

Excluding basal and squamous cell skin cancer, and carcinomas in situ, except urinary bladder. American Cancer Society, Surveillance Research, 1999.

Typically, prostate cancer grows slowly and remains confined to the prostate gland, where it doesn't cause any serious harm. But not all cancers act the same. Some forms of prostate cancer can be aggressive, and these aggressive cancers can quickly spread to other parts of the body.

What causes prostate cancer and why some types behave differently are unknown. Research suggests a combination of factors may play a role, including family history, ethnicity, hormones, diet and environment (see page 7).

However, this much is clear: Most men with prostate cancer that's detected while the cancer is still confined to the prostate gland can be cured. It's after the cancer has spread to nearby organs that treating the disease becomes more difficult — but not impossible.

Symptoms that may signal cancer

The problem with prostate cancer is that it often doesn't produce any symptoms in its early stages, when it's the easiest to treat. That's why approximately 40 percent of prostate cancers aren't diagnosed until they've spread beyond the prostate.

When symptoms do develop, they may be much like those you would experience with benign prostatic hyperplasia (BPH). You also may feel a dull pain in your lower pelvic area that doesn't subside. Your symptoms may include:

- A sudden need to urinate
- Difficulty starting to urinate
- Pain during urination
- Weak urine flow and dribbling
- Starting and stopping of your urine flow
- A sensation that your bladder isn't empty
- Frequent urination at night
- Blood in your urine
- Painful ejaculation
- General pain in the lower back, hips or upper thighs
- Loss of appetite and weight

How prostate cancer is diagnosed

A digital rectal exam and the prostate-specific antigen (PSA) test
are usually the first steps in diagnosing prostate cancer. If the
results of one or both tests are abnormal and your doctor suspects
cancer, he or she will have you undergo a biopsy. Analyzing small
tissue samples from the gland is the most effective way to tell if
you have prostate cancer.

To do a biopsy, your doctor will insert an ultrasound probe into
your rectum. Guided by images from the probe identifying suspect
areas, your doctor aims a fine, hollow needle at the center of the
prostate. Called a biopsy gun, this needle is powered by a spring
that instantly propels and retrieves a very thin section of tissue.

Occasionally, the biopsy needle is inserted into your prostate
through the perineum, the area between the anus and the scrotum.
More often, it's directed alongside the ultrasound probe and
inserted through the rectum.

Ordinarily, at least six sections of tissue are taken from different
areas of your prostate gland (sextant biopsy). Most of the samples
are taken from the outer area of your gland (peripheral zone),
where most cancers start. Sometimes, samples are taken from the
inner portion of the gland (transitional zone).

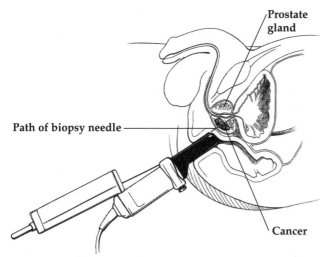

**During a biopsy, a thin needle is inserted into suspect areas and small sections of tissue
are retrieved for analysis.**

A biopsy can be painful, but most often it causes only minor discomfort because the needle used is very thin. Most people don't need anesthesia or sedatives during the procedure, or pain medication afterward. However, you will be given an enema. This reduces the risk of infection from digestive bacteria that might otherwise enter the needle incision. Antibiotics taken before and after the biopsy also further reduce the possibility of infection.

Common side effects of a biopsy include a small amount of rectal bleeding and blood in your urine for 1 to 2 days. Blood may appear in your semen, giving it a pink tint, for weeks to months afterward.

The tissue samples taken from your prostate are sent to a pathologist who specializes in diagnosing cancer and other tissue abnormalities. From the samples, the pathologist can tell if it's cancer and how aggressive the cancer is.

The biopsy samples also can identify specific cells that put you at significant risk of having cancer in the future. Known as prostatic intraepithelial neoplasia (PIN) these are abnormal cells that are in the early stage of becoming cancerous. If PIN is found, your doctor may recommend additional biopsies every 3 to 6 months for at least 2 years, depending on how abnormal the cells appear.

About half the men with more severe (high-grade) PIN have cancer by the next biopsy. If you have less severe (lower-grade) PIN and show no change after 2 years, your doctor may suggest reducing the frequency of biopsies to one each year.

Grading the cancer

When a biopsy confirms the presence of cancer, the next step, called grading, is to determine if it's a slow- or fast-growing form. A pathologist studies your prostate tissue samples on a series of slides under the microscope, comparing the cancer cells with healthy prostate cells. The more different the cancer cells are from the healthy cells, the more aggressive the cancer and the more likely it is to spread quickly.

Throughout the samples, cancer cells may vary in shape and size. Some cells may be aggressive, while others aren't. The pathologist identifies the two most prominent types of cancer cells when assigning a grade.

Cancers are graded on several kinds of scales. The most common scale runs from 1 to 5, with 1 being the least aggressive form of cancer and 5 being the most dangerous. The scale is named after pathologist Donald Gleason, M.D., who devised it.

Grade 1. The cells are small, shaped much alike and evenly spaced, similar to healthy cells.

Grade 2. The cells are more varied in size and shape, and more loosely scattered.

Grade 3. The cells are even more varied in size and shape, with some cells fused together into large, oddly shaped clumps that are scattered about.

Grade 4. Many cells are fused into strange-looking masses that are scattered haphazardly and invading nearby tissue.

Grade 5. Most of the cells have gathered into large, scattered masses that have invaded nearby tissues and organs.

The type of cancer that's most numerous in your biopsy gets one of these five grades. The cancer that's second most numerous also is given a grade. For example, your primary grade of cancer could be a 1, while your secondary grade of cancer is a 2. These two numbers are added together to determine a total Gleason score — in this case, 3.

The lower the score the better. Scores between 2 and 4 mean the cancer is growing slowly. Scores in the middle, between 5 and 7, can mean the cancer is slow- or fast-growing, depending on a

Interpreting the grades

Studies suggest that if you have a Gleason score of 2 to 4, there's about a 25 percent chance that your cancer will spread beyond your prostate in 10 years, where it can damage other organs and affect your survival. The likelihood doubles to a 50 percent chance with a Gleason score of 5 to 7. It triples to 75 percent with a Gleason score of 8 to 10.

variety of factors, including how long you've had the cancer. Scores at the high end of the scale, from 8 to 10, mean the cancer is fast-growing.

Has the cancer spread?

This determination is crucial, because cancer confined to the prostate has a high cure rate. Once the cancer extends beyond the prostate, the survival rate declines. To find out if your cancer has spread, you'll need to have more tests. Depending on your doctor and the type of cancer you have, you may undergo one or more of the following procedures:

Ultrasound
In addition to helping detect the presence of cancer, ultrasound can show if the cancer has invaded nearby tissues.

Bone scan
This is the most common test, because it can show the spread of cancer to bone better than any other procedure. Beforehand, a harmless, low-grade radioactive solution is injected into your bloodstream. This is a tracer solution that the bone scan will pick up plainly in a full-body skeletal image. The solution travels throughout your body like a heat-seeking missile and attaches itself to areas of new bone growth that may stem from cancer or from fractures, arthritis or infections.

During the scan, you lie on an examination table beneath a scanner. Your skeleton is displayed on a video monitor, with areas of rapid growth lighting up as "hot spots." Actually, these spots appear dark on the picture.

Interpreting the bone scan can be difficult in some people because the scan picks up more than cancer. However, doctors know that prostate cancer tends to spread first to bones near the prostate, such as the hips and lower spine. Also, isolated hot spots are more typical of cancer than a scan that shows corresponding hot spots on both sides of the body, such as arthritis in your right and left hips.

Chest X-ray

An X-ray film will show if the cancer has spread to your lungs. Though less than 5 percent of prostate cancer spreads this far, lung cancer will develop in about 25 percent of people with advanced prostate cancer.

CT scan

A computerized tomography (CT) scan produces three-dimensional, cross-sectional images of your body tissues that are stacked together on a computer screen, allowing a doctor to view specific parts of your body from any angle.

Before the CT scan, an iodine-based solution is injected into your bloodstream. This provides enhanced contrast to the X-ray images for clearer pictures. You may feel a temporary rush of heat as the solution spreads throughout your body, but you'll experience no pain. It's possible to do a CT without the iodine if you're allergic to the solution, but the pictures won't be as clear.

Here's how a CT scan works: You lie on a table that slowly glides through the middle of a large donut-shaped scanner. While you're lying down, the scanner takes a series of pictures showing different "slices" of tissue in the area of your prostate. The process may take up to 30 minutes.

A computer then stacks the image slices together to form a detailed picture of your prostate and the area surrounding it. In addition to cancer, a CT scan can identify enlarged lymph nodes. When cancer begins to spread, one of the first places it goes to is your lymph nodes. The lymph nodes trap and try to destroy abnormal cells, causing the nodes to swell and become overwhelmed by the cancer.

Unfortunately, CT can identify only lymph nodes that look abnormal, not those with microscopic levels of cancer. Your lymph nodes may be swollen for other reasons. Therefore, CT is most useful only when combined with other tests.

MRI

Like a CT scan, magnetic resonance imaging (MRI) produces a detailed, three-dimensional picture of your body. Its primary value in the diagnosis of prostate cancer is to detect the spread of cancer to lymph nodes and bone.

Instead of using X-rays and dyes to generate the pictures, MRI uses magnetic and radio waves. A radiofrequency pulse passes through your body, generating a current that is picked up on a radiofrequency receiver and is then translated into a picture that looks much like a CT image.

During MRI, you lie inside a small, tube-shaped device for 30 to 45 minutes. It's not painful, but the machine makes noises, like those of a woodpecker, and some people get anxious when enclosed in the small space. If this might be a problem for you, a sedative beforehand can help calm you.

Because of the more sophisticated equipment involved, an MRI is more expensive than a CT scan. That's why it's not as commonly used as CT.

Lymph node biopsy

The best way to determine if the cancer has spread to nearby lymph nodes is with a lymphadenectomy (lim-FAD-uh-NEK-tuh-mee). During this procedure, some of the nodes near the prostate are removed and examined under a microscope.

If other tests, such as a bone or CT scan, show that the cancer has spread, then a lymphadenectomy usually isn't necessary. The procedure is most often used to confirm the results of tests indicating that the cancer is confined to the prostate.

There are two ways to remove lymph nodes:

Laparoscopic surgery. Following general anesthesia, a surgeon makes a couple of tiny incisions in your abdomen. With a long surgical instrument that contains a tiny fiber-optic camera (laparoscope), lymph nodes in your pelvic area are removed and sent to a pathologist for analysis.

Traditional surgery. Once you've been anesthetized, a surgeon makes about a 3-inch incision between your navel and pubic area, and then locates and removes the lymph nodes through the incision. This method is most often done if your doctor is planning to do surgery to remove the prostate gland but wants to confirm beforehand that the cancer hasn't spread beyond the prostate.

Prostate cancer progression

T1a
Cancer found during
another procedure; equals 5%
or less of removed tissue

T1b
Cancer found during
another procedure; equals
more than 5% of removed tissue

T1c
Cancer detected by high
PSA level; cannot be felt

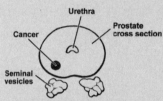

T2a
Cancer confined to
half or less of one lobe

T2b
Cancer occupies more
than half of one lobe

T2c
Cancer found in
both lobes

T3a
Cancer growing
outside of one lobe

T3b
Cancer growing
outside of both lobes

T3c
Cancer spread to one
or both seminal vesicles

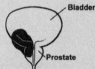

T4a
Cancer spread to
bladder neck, external
sphincter and/or rectum

T4b
Cancer spread to
other nearby tissues

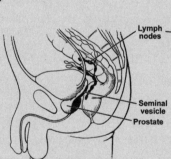

N1-3
Cancer spread to
nearby lymph nodes

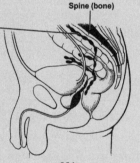

M1
Cancer spread beyond
prostate region to bones,
liver, lungs, etc.

Staging the cancer

Once all of your diagnostic tests are complete, your doctor will use the results of the tests to assign a stage to the cancer. This designation communicates to other health care personnel how advanced the cancer is.

Some men find staging information helpful in understanding the severity of their disease, and in discussing possible treatment options with their doctor. Other men find the information a little overwhelming. The important point is that if you have questions about your diagnosis or cancer stage, that you discuss them with your doctor.

Most doctors use one of two staging systems:

TNM system

This is the most popular method in the United States for identifying the progression of cancer. When the pathologist sends your doctor a report that stages your cancer, the report will include three capital letters — T, N and M.

- T stands for tumor and signifies the extent of the cancer in, and adjacent to, the prostate gland.
- N stands for nodes (lymph nodes) and signifies whether the cancer has, or has not, spread to nearby lymph nodes.
- M stands for metastasis (muh-TAS-tuh-sis), the medical term for cancer that has spread to other tissues or organs, such as bone or the lungs.

The three letters are followed by a number and perhaps another letter in small type. The numbers range from 0 to 4 and represent the extent of the tumor. The small letters go from a to c and indicate the location of the cancer.

Once the T, N and M results are known, the cancer is then assigned one of four stages based on the findings (see "TNM stage groupings"on the following page).

Stage I. It signifies very early cancer that's confined to micro-scopic particles that cannot be felt.

Stage II. The cancer can be felt but it remains confined to the prostate gland.

TNM stage groupings	
Stage I	T1, N0, M0
Stage II	T2, N0, M0
Stage III	T3, N0, M0
Stage IV	T4, N0, M0; Any T, N1-3, M0; Any T, any N, M1

Stage III. The cancer has spread beyond the prostate to the seminal vesicles or nearby bladder tissues.

Stage IV. This represents advanced cancer that has spread to lymph nodes, bones, lungs or other organs.

ABCD system

Some doctors use this older and more traditional cancer staging system, in which A and B represent cancer that's confined to the prostate gland, and C and D indicate cancer that has spread to other parts of the body.

Like the TNM system, each capital letter in the ABCD system is followed by a subcategory that represents details in the staging. Because the ABCD system has fewer categories available, it's slightly less precise.

Survival statistics

Survival rates for prostate cancer have improved considerably in the past two decades. In the early 1980s, a diagnosis of prostate cancer meant you had a 63 percent chance of living 5 years. Today, you have a 93 percent chance of living 5 years. About 68 percent of men with prostate cancer live 10 years, and 52 percent live 15 years or more.

Hopefully, survival figures will continue to improve if more men have regular digital rectal exams and PSA tests to identify cancer during early stages, when it can be cured. For cancer that's caught early and confined to the prostate, the survival rate is almost 100 percent.

Answers to your questions

What are tumor markers?
These are substances made from cancerous cells found in blood.
When they exist in elevated levels, they may indicate the presence
of cancer. During treatment and follow-up visits, your blood may
be routinely checked for elevated tumor markers. PSA is a tumor
marker for prostate cancer.

Is a biopsy the only way I can be sure I have prostate cancer?
Yes. Other tests, such as a rectal exam or PSA test, can suggest a
strong possibility of prostate cancer. But a biopsy is the only way to
be certain.

Can a biopsy be wrong?
When tissue samples are taken from the gland, it's possible to miss
the cancer. This is called a sampling error. A biopsy result that
comes back normal isn't a guarantee that you don't have cancer.
Sampling errors, however, are uncommon.

Can a biopsy loosen cancer cells, allowing them to spread?
No evidence suggests that this can happen. Cancer cells not
removed in the biopsy stay within the tumor where they have
been growing.

Why do I need to stop taking aspirin before a biopsy?
Aspirin and some other pain medications "thin" your blood and
can increase your risk of bleeding. Discontinuing these medications
for a short period before and after a prostate biopsy will reduce
your chances of serious bleeding from the procedure. The same is
true for prescription blood-thinners taken to reduce clotting, such
as warfarin (Coumadin).

Is it possible for a biopsy to cause impotence?
No. Impotence that follows a biopsy is probably due to stress that
often accompanies cancer diagnosis and treatment. In some cases it
may result from temporary inflammation.

Can I pass cancer on to my wife during sexual intercourse?
No. Cancer cells won't escape from your body through intercourse. Even if they could, they wouldn't be able to grow inside another person because they're genetically coded for your body.

Chapter 7

What Are Your Options?

Finding out you have cancer can lead to panic. You may feel as if you need to make an instant decision and begin your treatment right away. However, because prostate cancer is often a slow-growing cancer, there's generally no need to rush.

Give yourself a little time to gather some information and consider your treatment options. You may want to visit the patient education library, if your medical center has one. Or you can stop at your local library, or check out well-respected sources on the Internet, such as the American Cancer Society or American Urological Association. Once you've read up on your condition, write down questions you want to ask your doctor before the two of you decide on a treatment plan.

You also may find it helpful to take a family member or friend with you to your next appointment. He or she can remind you of important questions you want to ask. That person also can listen intently and help you recall the discussion afterward, including important points made.

Often, there's more than one way to treat prostate cancer, and you might even use a "one-two punch," a combination of treatments such as surgery followed by radiation. Which treatment you and your doctor choose will depend on several factors, such as how fast-growing the cancer is, how much it has spread, your age, and your health, as well as the benefits and potential side effects of the treatment.

Letting the cancer alone

Because blood tests can now detect prostate cancer at a very early stage, more men are being given an option that's less traumatic than traditional treatments. It goes by many names, such as "watchful waiting," "observation" or "expectant therapy." You do nothing except keep a close watch on the cancer with regular blood tests and rectal exams, performed about every 6 months. You may also need to have occasional biopsies.

If you're fairly young and healthy, in your 50s or 60s, your doctor probably won't recommend this approach. Because of your age, the cancer has many years to grow, and even a small, slow-growing cancer might eventually reach the point when it needs additional treatment. The cancer cells could also unexpectedly become aggressive and spread so much that a cure becomes difficult or impossible.

However, if you're age 70 or older and the cancer is small and slow-growing, watchful waiting might be an option. Chances are good that without any form of treatment, you'll live 10 more years without the cancer spreading, or without it causing you problems. With careful monitoring, you'd be able to act quickly if the cancer did turn aggressive, and treatment became necessary to stop its growth.

Are you a candidate for watchful waiting?
- You're age 70 or older with a small, low-grade cancer (Gleason score of 2 to 4).
- The cancer is confined to the prostate and you want time to think about your options.
- You aren't able to withstand the side effects of treatment for age or health reasons.
- Your future life expectancy is less than 10 years, because of another condition.

What are the benefits?
- You avoid the risks associated with other treatments, such as impotence or incontinence.

- Watchful waiting buys you time to consider treatment options. It can take several years for a tiny tumor to double in size, and you can use this time to your benefit.
- It's the least expensive option, requiring only occasional exams and tests.

What are the disadvantages?

- The cancer can grow while you wait. Though rare, a slow-growing cancer can turn into a faster-growing cancer in weeks to months. Among men with a Gleason score of 2 to 4, about 2 percent develop cancer outside the prostate within the first year.
- You may become the "walking worried," always anxious about your cancer and preoccupied with your tests and condition. Though more aggressive treatment has risks, it reduces the fear that you may be gambling with your life.

Removing your prostate gland

The surest way to cure cancer that's confined to your prostate gland is to remove the gland. This type of surgery is called radical prostatectomy.

Until a few years ago, a radical prostatectomy just about guaranteed devastating consequences: Nearly every man who had this procedure became impotent or suffered from diminished sexual function. Many men had bladder problems. In addition, most men had so much blood loss during the surgery that they needed transfusions.

New procedures and instruments developed during the past two decades have changed this surgery drastically. Surgeons now use special techniques to cut free the prostate, while sparing muscles and attached nerve bundles that control urination and sexual function. Methods to control heavy bleeding are now routine.

Because of these refinements, 1 in 4 men with prostate cancer now choose surgery. A decade ago, only 1 in 10 chose surgery.

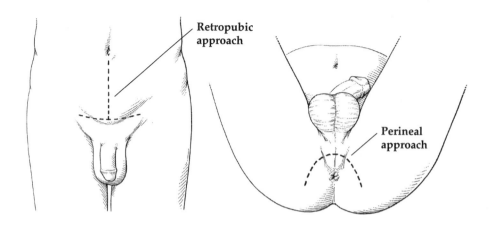

Retropubic approach

Perineal approach

With retropubic surgery, the prostate gland is removed through an incision in the lower abdomen. Perineal surgery involves removing the gland through an incision between the anus and the scrotal sac.

Retropubic surgery

Retropubic surgery is one of two methods for removing the prostate. In this procedure, the gland is taken out through an incision in the lower abdomen that typically runs from just below the navel to an inch above the penis (see illustration).

It's the most common form of prostate removal for two reasons: The surgeon can use the same incision to remove surrounding lymph nodes, which are tested to make sure the cancer hasn't spread. In addition, the procedure gives the surgeon better access to the prostate, making it easier to save the nerve bundles that control erection.

The night before surgery you'll likely be given an enema or laxatives to clear your rectum of any fecal matter. This reduces the chance of infection if the rectal wall is punctured during surgery, an uncommon but possible risk.

You may choose to be put to sleep during the surgery with general anesthesia, or have an epidural injection that numbs only the lower half of your body. General anesthesia is more common.

After the incision, the surgeon may remove lymph nodes near your prostate and send the sample to a pathologist. Enlarged or suspect lymph nodes can be evaluated by frozen-section techniques to determine if cancer is present. Results are often known within 15 to 30 minutes. If cancer is found, your surgeon may close the incision without removing the gland, or may proceed with the surgery. The decision to proceed in light of positive lymph nodes depends on the number of lymph nodes involved, your age, and associated symptoms. The fewer nodes that contain cancer, the younger your age, and the fewer symptoms you have, the more likely your doctor will be to continue with surgery.

Once the prostate is removed, the surgeon will reconstruct part of your bladder, attaching the urethra and the sphincter muscle located below the site of the now-removed prostate directly to the bladder. This procedure increases your chances of being able to control your flow of urine, though it may take weeks, possibly even several months, for your body to heal enough for you to regain bladder control.

Depending on where the cancer is, your surgeon will try to save the nerve bundles attached to each side of the prostate. These nerves control your ability to have an erection. Surgeons can often spare one or both of these bundles if the cancer isn't too close.

Men in their 40s and 50s who have this nerve-sparing surgery are more likely to retain their ability to have an erection than older men. For some older men — especially those not sexually active — the spared nerves don't survive the shock of surgery. On average, half of men who are sexually active before surgery experience impotence or diminished sexual functioning, such as loss of orgasm or reduced sensation, after surgery. For men who already are impotent at the time of surgery, the nerve bundles are generally removed because they're no longer needed and there's a remote chance they could contain some cancer cells.

If even one nerve bundle is spared, it's still possible to have erections. However, because the prostate and seminal vesicles produce most of the seminal fluid, after surgery your ejaculations will contain very little fluid. If neither nerve bundle can be spared, you can still have a normal sex drive (libido) and orgasms, though without normal erections. Chapter 10 discusses devices and medications that can help you achieve an erection if you can no longer do so naturally.

After surgery, recovery in the hospital for 1 to 3 days, and 3 to 5 weeks at home, is typical. You'll also need to use a catheter for about 2 to 3 weeks to give your urinary tract time to heal.

Perineal surgery
With this form of surgery, an incision is made between the anus and the scrotal sac holding the testicles. There's generally less bleeding with perineal surgery, and heavier men recover sooner. Unfortunately, this approach makes it much more difficult — and sometimes impossible — for your surgeon to locate and save the nerve bundles attached to the prostate. In addition, the surgeon isn't able to reach nearby lymph nodes. That's why this surgery is less commonly used.

Are you a candidate for surgery?
- Your cancer is confined to the prostate.
- You're healthy enough to withstand surgery.
- Your expected life span is greater than the cancer would let you live.

What are the benefits?
For cancer that's confined to the prostate gland, surgery is the most effective treatment. It can cure your disease.

What are the disadvantages?
- All surgery carries some risk. Though the mortality rate is low, approximately 1 percent of men who have surgery die as a result of complications. Your risk increases with your age.
- You may become impotent. This depends a lot on your age. Between 60 percent and 80 percent of men younger than age 50 who have nerve-sparing surgery are able to achieve normal erections afterward. For men in their 70s, only about 15 percent to 25 percent maintain normal sexual functioning. The skill of your surgeon and the quality of your erections before surgery can affect the outcome. If you had trouble achieving or maintaining an erection before surgery, the chances are greater that you'll be impotent after surgery.

- You may experience incontinence — at least temporarily. After the catheter is removed, nearly all men have some bladder-control problems for at least a few days. You could have problems for weeks, or even months. If so, medications and treatment can help improve bladder control. About 95 percent of men eventually regain complete control. Most of the remainder experience "stress" incontinence, meaning they can't hold their urine flow when pressure is placed on the bladder, as happens when you sneeze, cough, laugh or lift.
- Recovery can take 1 to 2 months.
- There's a small risk of damage to your lower intestine or rectum. More surgery may be necessary to repair the damage.

Destroying the cancer with radiation

Radiation treatment uses high-powered X-rays or other radiation to kill cancer cells. It's generally the preferred treatment if you're older or in poor health and might have a hard time withstanding surgery. For cancer confined to the prostate, radiation is often as effective as surgery for as much as 10 years.

Radiation also is used to treat cancer that has spread outside your prostate. It can destroy cancerous cells, shrink tumors and relieve painful symptoms.

External beam
Radiation is most commonly delivered by a beam from a large machine placed over your body. Unfortunately, these "external beams" do more than destroy cancerous cells. They can damage healthy tissue in the same area.

That's why the first step in radiation therapy is to map out the areas in your body to receive radiation. Three-dimensional scans show the location of the prostate and surrounding organs. Computer imaging software allows a radiation therapist to rotate the picture in any direction to find the best angles to fire the beams.

Treatments are generally given 5 days a week for about 6 or 7 weeks. Each treatment takes about 15 minutes. However, much of this is preparation time. The actual length of time you receive radiation is only about 1 minute. To make sure the beams are always precisely on the mark, you'll have a body supporter that will hold you in the same position for each treatment. You'll also be asked to arrive with a full bladder, which will help hold your prostate in the same position during each treatment. Ink marks on your skin will help the radiation therapist hit the same targets each time. Custom-designed shields cover nearby areas such as your intestines, anus, rectal wall and urethra, protecting them from scattered rays.

During the procedure, you'll lie on a table while a machine known as a linear accelerator moves above you, targeting the cancer with radiation. The first phase of treatment usually involves blanketing the entire pelvic region with low doses of radiation to kill any microscopic cancer cells that have wandered away from detectable tumors. This continues for about 2 weeks.

During the second phase of treatment, the beams generally are narrowed and strengthened to target individual tumors. This gives your intestines and bladder a rest from the radiation. Higher doses of radiation are more effective in killing cancer, but they're also more damaging to healthy tissue. After about 2 weeks of targeting the tumors, you may receive another 2 weeks or so of blanket radiation throughout your pelvis.

A new and promising external beam therapy uses protons instead of X-rays to kill the cancer. Protons are parts of atoms that cause little damage to surrounding tissue but effectively destroy cells at the end of the beam. The protons travel through noncancerous tissues and come to rest in the targeted area, where they deposit their radiation dose. This allows your therapist to deliver stronger doses of beam radiation.

Seed implants

A second radiation method that's gaining popularity uses ultrasound-guided needles to inject rice-size radioactive seeds into your prostate (see illustration). These seeds deliver double the dose of radiation of external beams, and the seeds cause less damage to healthy tissue.

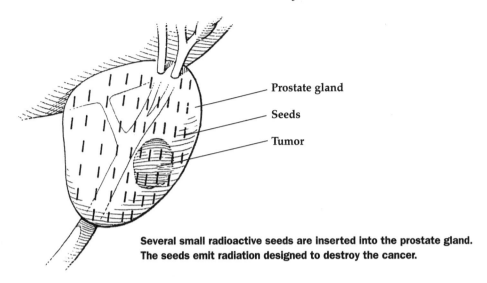

Prostate gland

Seeds

Tumor

Several small radioactive seeds are inserted into the prostate gland. The seeds emit radiation designed to destroy the cancer.

The procedure takes about an hour and is done on an outpatient basis, with either general anesthesia or spinal (epidural) anesthesia that numbs the lower portion of your body.

Between 70 and 150 rice-size seeds are inserted throughout your prostate by way of a needle that passes through the skin of your perineum, the area between your scrotum and anus. The number of seeds inserted depends on the size of your prostate. The therapy generally works better on smaller or moderate-sized prostates.

Radioactive seeds may contain one of several radioactive substances, depending on the grade of the cancer. Typically, you'll be given iodine if your Gleason score is less than 6, or the more potent palladium (puh-LAY-de-um) if your score is higher. These seeds are left in even after they stop emitting radiation. Other seeds that contain an even more potent substance, called iridium (i-RID-ee-um), are left in only temporarily.

An ultrasound probe inserted into your rectum guides the doctor in placing the seeds throughout your prostate, without missing any areas. A template attached to the outside of the probe and held up against your perineum guides and steadies the needles loaded with seeds.

Iodine and palladium seeds generally emit radiation only a few millimeters beyond where they're implanted. Although this type of radiation isn't thought to escape your prostate area, doctors recommend that for the first couple of months you stay at least 6 feet away from children and pregnant women, who are especially sensitive to radiation. Within a year, all radiation inside the pellets is generally exhausted.

Because seed implantation is new, its long-term effects are unknown. But encouraging short-term results suggest that this could become a common form of prostate cancer therapy in the decade ahead. According to early studies, radioactive seeds control cancer growth for 5 years in 90 percent of men, and for 10 years in 85 percent of men. In 2 out of 3 men, the seeds destroy the cancer.

Seed implants generally produce fewer side effects than external beam radiation. Impotence occurs in about 1 out of 6 men, compared with 1 in 2 for beam radiation. Incontinence is rare.

Are you a candidate for radiation?
- Your cancer can't be cured by surgery because it has spread outside the prostate.
- Your cancer is confined to the prostate and is a low- or medium-grade.
- You don't want surgery.
- You expect to live longer than your cancer would allow you to live.

What are the benefits?
- For cancer confined to the prostate, radiation is nearly as effective as surgery over a 10-year period.
- The procedure is generally done on an outpatient basis. With seed implantation, you may need to spend one night in the hospital.
- Radiation doesn't entail the trauma and recovery associated with surgery.

What are the disadvantages?
- Radiation can affect your sexual function. Over time, it can damage the nerves that control erections and the arteries that carry blood to your penis. Most men don't have problems with erections or intercourse in the early months after radiation

therapy. But eventually most men suffer some complications. Only about half of men who had normal sexual function before radiation retain it after therapy. The percentage is higher for seed implantation therapy. The younger you are, the better your chance of retaining the ability to have normal sexual relations.

- Beam therapy can sap your energy and appetite. Both should return within a couple of months after treatment.

- Some men have intestinal problems from external beam therapy, including nausea, diarrhea, rectal bleeding, a burning feeling around the anus, and a sense that you need to have a bowel movement. The symptoms generally subside when the treatments are over. But for about 5 percent of men, they continue.

- Beam therapy produces urinary problems in approximately 3 out of 4 men. The most common complaints are constantly feeling as if you have to urinate, blood in your urine, painful urination with a burning sensation, and urine leakage. About 5 percent of men experience severe symptoms and need to be hospitalized. Less than 1 percent of those hospitalized require surgery to correct the problem.

Freezing cancer cells (cryotherapy)

Another way to kill prostate cancer is to freeze the prostate — almost like turning it into an iceball. Doctors use a similar approach to kill warts, dipping a swab into a tank of supercooled liquid nitrogen, then dabbing the swab onto the wart, which eventually dies and falls off. Prostate tissue dies in the same way and is absorbed and then eliminated by your body.

Called cryotherapy, the procedure involves inserting 5 to 7 thin metal rods, each about 6 inches long, through the perineum and into the prostate. An ultrasound probe in the rectum helps your doctor position the rods. Once the rod tips are in place, liquid nitrogen is released into the rods, where it circulates and plunges the temperature to about -374 F. As the tissue freezes, the formation and expansion of ice crystals within the cancerous cells cause them to rupture and die. To keep the urethra from freezing along with your prostate, a catheter is placed inside the urethra and filled with a warming solution.

The entire procedure takes about 2 hours, with most of the time used to carefully position the rods and about 30 minutes to freeze the prostate.

You can expect to stay in the hospital 1 to 2 days. You'll probably be able to return to your normal activities in a couple of weeks. However, it will take your body about 9 months to a year to shed the dead cells. The procedure may have to be repeated.

Are you a candidate for cryotherapy?
- Your cancer is confined to the prostate.
- You're not healthy enough to withstand surgery or radiation.
- You don't want surgery or radiation.

What are the advantages?
- Cryotherapy controls cancer confined to the prostate in about 80 percent of men.

---

10 questions to ask your doctor

To help determine the best form of treatment for you, ask your doctor these questions:

1. What options are available to me?
2. How fast will the cancer grow if left untreated?
3. Do you think the cancer can be cured with treatment? If so, what are the chances?
4. Which treatment would you recommend, and why?
5. How many times have you performed this procedure?
6. How soon before we know if the treatment has worked?
7. What are my risks of lasting side effects, such as impotence or incontinence?
8. How soon will I be able to return to work?
9. Will I have to restrict any activities?
10. If the treatment doesn't work, do I have another option?

- The procedure requires only 1 or 2 days in the hospital and can sometimes be done on an outpatient basis.
- There's very little blood loss.
- Recovery time is short, just 1 or 2 weeks.

What are the disadvantages?
- The procedure is fairly new and not widely used.
- Cryotherapy doesn't always kill all the cancer cells on the first try. It may have to be repeated.
- You have a 90 percent chance of impotence developing. The nerve bundles that control erections can freeze and die.
- You may have trouble urinating for several weeks afterward. The freezing makes the prostate temporarily swell, which squeezes the urethra.
- You'll have temporary bruising and soreness where the rods are inserted.
- Though the short-term results look encouraging, long-term survival rates appear lower than with surgery or radiation.

Answers to your questions

Is surgery more difficult in some men?
Radical prostatectomy can be more challenging in men who are obese or who have an especially deep or narrow pelvis. A very large prostate also can be more challenging to remove. However, a skilled surgeon should be able to overcome these obstacles.

Isn't radiation harmful?
Uncontrolled amounts of radiation can be dangerous, even deadly. The amount you receive during radiation therapy is precisely calculated and controlled to cause only minimal damage to healthy cells.

Can the radioactive seeds work their way out of the prostate gland?
Occasionally some seeds can get into the urethra and be excreted in your urine. This generally doesn't cause problems.

Should I get a second opinion before making a decision?
Again, that depends. If you feel confident in your doctor and comfortable with your treatment plan, a second opinion may not be necessary. However, if you have some concerns about your diagnosis, you don't feel confident in your doctor, or you don't feel comfortable with the treatment he or she is recommending, then it may be advisable to get another opinion.

Chapter 8

When the Cancer Is Advanced

For cancer that has spread outside the prostate gland, curing the disease becomes more difficult. However, certain treatments can help slow its growth and even shrink the tumors. This means an opportunity for you to live longer and enjoy a better quality of life, even though you may have advanced cancer.

Controlling the cancer with hormones

Many prostate cancers feed off androgens — from the Greek words *andros* (man) and *gennan* (to produce). These male sex hormones produce male characteristics. Testosterone, the main male sex hormone, is responsible for the normal development of sex organs and other male features, such as facial hair and large muscles.

When you have prostate cancer, the circulation of male sex hormones throughout your body and around the cancer makes the cancer grow faster. The most common way to treat advanced prostate cancer is to cut off the supply of these hormones to the cancer. About 75 percent of men with advanced prostate cancer choose this form of treatment. Hormone therapy uses drugs to do one or two things, sometimes both:

- Stop your body from producing most, but not all, male sex hormones
- Block remaining hormones from getting into cancer cells

Hormone therapy is so effective at shrinking tumors that it's being used in some early-stage cancers, too, in combination with surgery and radiation. The hormones shrink large tumors so that surgery or radiation can destroy them more easily. And after surgery or radiation, the drugs can help kill stray cells left behind at the tumor site.

In one study, 79 percent of the men who had both radiation and hormone therapy were still alive after 5 years, compared with 62 percent of the men who received only radiation.

There are three different types of hormone therapy:

Drugs that decrease testosterone production

More than 90 percent of testosterone is produced by the testicles. One popular hormone treatment sets up a chemical blockade, preventing the testicles from receiving messages to make testosterone. These messages initially come from the hypothalamus, an area of your brain that secretes chemicals to control many body functions. One of these chemicals is luteinizing-hormone-releasing hormone (LHRH). It alerts the pituitary gland, located just below your brain, to release luteinizing hormone (LH), the chemical that signals your testicles to make testosterone.

Several medications known as LHRH agonists can interrupt this message pathway. The medications are synthetic hormones similar to your brain's natural LHRH. But instead of turning on the chemical switch that activates LH, they turn it off. Your testicles never get the message to produce testosterone.

Two of the more common LHRH blockers are leuprolide (Lupron) and goserelin (Zoladex). They're injected into your buttocks once every 3 months for the rest of your life.

Drugs that block the ability to use your hormones

Not all testosterone is produced in the testicles. Around 5 percent to 10 percent comes from the adrenal glands, located above each of your kidneys. Medications known as antiandrogens keep this form of testosterone away from the cancer cells.

The drugs compete with testosterone for entrance into the cancer cells, eventually crowding out the testosterone. Three drugs, which come in tablet form, are most frequently used, flutamide (Eulexin), bicalutamide (Casodex) and nilutamide (Nilandron). Depending on the brand of drug you're prescribed, you take the medication one to three times a day.

This therapy is often used in combination with LHRH drugs, causing little or no testosterone to get to the cancer cells. Doctors refer to the combination as total androgen blockade.

Intermittent drug use

Depriving prostate cancer of testosterone usually doesn't kill the cancer. Within 1 to 3 years, the cancer often becomes resistant and learns to thrive without testosterone. Once this happens, options to stop the cancer are limited.

Some researchers suspect continuous use of hormone medications may be the reason the cancer learns to adapt. These researchers believe that taking occasional breaks from the medication might keep the cancer from adjusting to the testosterone loss, or at least slow down the process. Clinical studies are now testing this idea.

Exactly how cancer cells become resistant is a mystery. There are many different kinds of prostate cancer cells. Two broad categories are "hormone-sensitive cancer cells" and "hormone-insensitive cancer cells." When you get prostate cancer, you probably have some of both. The more hormone-sensitive cells you have, the better you'll respond to hormone treatment. The fewer you have, the worse you'll respond. In time, the hormone-sensitive cells die, but the hormone-insensitive cells pick up the slack and grow unchecked.

With intermittent therapy, you stop taking hormone drugs after your PSA drops to a low level and remains steady. You resume the drugs after your PSA level rises again, generally above 10 nanograms per milliliter. During the drug-free periods, which can last a year or more, you aren't bothered by side effects of the medications, including decreased sex drive, impotence and breast enlargement.

Are you a candidate for hormone therapy?

Your cancer has spread outside the prostate gland.

What are the benefits?

- Hormone therapy can temporarily slow the growth of prostate cancer and shrink existing tumors, reducing your symptoms and allowing you to live longer.
- It's approximately 80 percent effective for 1 to 3 years.
- It can be stopped, allowing the return of normal hormone production.

What are the disadvantages?

- Hormone therapy lowers or eliminates the sex drive in most men.
- It often causes impotence.
- It can cause hot flushes, similar to those women often experience during menopause.
- It may cause your breasts to slightly enlarge and become sore. Low doses of radiation treatment can prevent this.
- It produces weight gain, often 10 to 15 pounds.
- It reduces your muscle and bone mass, making you more prone to broken bones.
- Some drugs cause nausea, diarrhea and fatigue.
- In rare cases it can lead to liver damage.
- Most cancers become resistant to the medication in 1 to 3 years.
- Some medications can cost hundreds of dollars a month and may not be covered by insurance.

With current hormone therapy, about 50 percent of men whose cancer has spread to other pelvic organs, such as the bladder and the rectum, live for 5 years. About 40 percent live for 10 years. If the cancer has spread to bone, time is often shortened. About 50 percent of men live 2 years. Approximately 30 percent live 5 years.

Choosing testicular surgery

Surgically removing the testicles to prevent testosterone production was once the standard treatment for advanced prostate cancer. It's still done occasionally, but hormone-blocking drugs have reduced the need for testicular surgery by providing what amounts to chemical castration.

Bilateral orchiectomy (OR-kee-EK-tuh-mee) is the medical term for testicle removal. "Orchi" is from the Greek word *orchis* meaning testicle, and "ectomy" means removal. "Bilateral" refers to the fact that both testicles are removed.

The procedure is often performed on an outpatient basis using a local anesthetic. The doctor will make a small incision at the center of your scrotum, the pouch that holds your testicles. Each testicle is clipped from the attached spermatic cord and removed. Most of the cord is left for a natural appearance. Some men have an artificial testicular implant placed into the scrotum during the surgery to maintain a more normal appearance.

Are you a candidate for orchiectomy?
- You can't tolerate hormone therapy for other health reasons.
- You aren't able to take daily medication as prescribed, or regularly visit the doctor's office for hormone injections.

What are the benefits?
- The procedure is quick and performed on an outpatient basis.
- The risk of complications is low.
- It's less expensive than hormone medications.
- Its effects are almost immediate. Within a few hours, the only testosterone left is the small amount coming from your adrenal glands.
- Men who select surgery tend to report a better quality of life than men who choose hormone injections. The side effects are generally less intense.

What are the disadvantages?
- It doesn't eliminate the 5 percent to 10 percent of the testosterone produced by the adrenal glands.
- As with hormone medications, the surgery reduces or eliminates the sex drive in most men.
- It leaves most men impotent.
- Half of the men experience breast enlargement or soreness.

- Approximately half of the men experience hot flushes.
- You may feel less masculine and become depressed, like the feelings a woman may have after breast removal or a hysterectomy.
- It can lead to osteoporosis, a disorder that weakens your bones and increases your risk of fractures.
- Though your cancer will probably go into remission for 1 to 3 years, it will almost certainly return, because the cancer cells adapt to the absence of hormones.

After testicular surgery, about 50 percent of men live 3 more years. About 25 percent live 5 years or more. Men with cancer confined to the pelvic area generally live even longer: 50 percent to 60 percent live 5 years, and 40 percent live 10 years or more.

Using chemotherapy

Chemotherapy is a first-line treatment for many forms of cancer, and is often tremendously effective at destroying cancer cells. Unfortunately, prostate cancer isn't among those cancers helped by chemotherapy. For this reason, it's generally used only as a last resort, usually after hormone therapy has failed.

As the name suggests, chemotherapy uses chemicals — anti-cancer drugs — to kill cancer cells. These drugs may be given intravenously, injected with a needle, or taken as pills. The main drawback of chemotherapy is the high rate of side effects. The drugs are toxic not only to cancer cells but to healthy cells. Chemotherapy can, for example, destroy infection-fighting white blood cells that make up your immune system, leaving you at high risk of infection from bacteria or a virus. Some drugs cause your hair to fall out, while others make you nauseated or sap your energy. The side effects usually end when the treatment ends.

Though chemotherapy has an unpopular history in the treatment of prostate cancer, this could change as researchers experiment with new cancer-fighting drugs. The drug suramin, for example, can destroy cells that are resistant to hormone therapy and also can block hormones released from the adrenal glands.

But the drug doesn't help everyone and can actually worsen the health of some men. Depending on the type of cancer cells you have, you may respond differently to chemotherapy from someone else who receives the same treatment. Researchers hope to identify certain chemotherapy drugs that destroy different types of cells when taken in combination.

Are you a candidate for chemotherapy?
Your cancer is resistant to hormone therapy and you don't want an orchiectomy.

What are the benefits?
- The medications may help reduce your pain.
- There's a slight possibility the medications may slow the growth of cancer cells.

What are the disadvantages?
- Chemotherapy has a dismal track record in helping men with prostate cancer. Current drugs don't appear to lengthen life.
- Side effects of the drugs can decrease your quality of life: You may experience nausea and vomiting, loss of appetite and energy, loss of hair, and mouth sores. One of the most dangerous side effects is the damage to your white blood cells, significantly increasing your risk of infection.

Trying an experimental procedure

If traditional treatments are unable to control the cancer, your doctor may suggest that you participate in an experimental therapy, also known as a clinical trial.

Experimental therapies don't involve rare drugs that researchers know little about. Only those treatments that show promise are tested on humans. Taking part in a clinical trial doesn't necessarily mean that your situation is hopeless. Your doctor may want you to try a particular new treatment because it shows signs of helping men with your specific health profile.

Gene therapy

One area of research that's still in its infancy but may offer hope for the future involves manipulation of human genes. Several promising possibilities are being tested.

Vaccines that boost your immune system. Your immune system is capable of attacking cancerous cells, but it often can't differentiate them from normal cells. Researchers are studying the possibility of removing prostate cancer cells and genetically altering the cells to make them more recognizable as foreign invaders. The altered cells are then injected back into your body to help your immune system recognize and destroy all prostate cancer cells. Experiments with animals show a 30 percent long-term cure rate after just three injections.

These vaccines are now being tested in humans. If they prove successful, they could one day be used not only to kill existing cancer, but to protect men at high risk of prostate cancer.

Drugs that block cancer-causing genes. Researchers have found that some prostate cancer involves a gene known as HER-2, which is usually associated with breast cancer. The bioengineered drug trastuzumab (Herceptin), which blocks HER-2 growth in late-stage breast cancer, may be helpful in some men.

Genetic changes in chromosomes 8, 10, 16 and 17 also are linked to prostate cancer. Researchers are attempting to identify the individual genes involved, in the hope of suppressing them.

Genes that alter cancer cells. One experimental approach uses genes that link with cancer cells, making the cancer vulnerable to drugs that wouldn't normally affect it. For instance, when the HSVtk gene comes into contact with a prostate tumor, this gene renders the tumor cells susceptible to the drug ganciclovir (Cytovene), used to treat herpes.

Genes that seek out and destroy cancer cells. This idea, still in the theory stage, involves injecting toxic genes into the body, which are coded to switch on only when they come into contact with prostate cancer cells, limiting damage to healthy cells.

To find out more about clinical studies taking place, ask your doctor or contact a cancer organization, such as the National Cancer Institute (see page 168).

Strategies for relieving pain

Early-stage prostate cancer typically isn't painful. However, once the cancer spreads beyond the gland to nearby bone, it may produce intense pain. This pain isn't something you need to live with. There are many effective methods for relieving the difficult pain of cancer.

Treating local pain

If you experience pain in a specific area of your body, such as your lower back, you have these options for treating it:

Spot radiation. It's similar to external beam radiation therapy, but instead of targeting known tumors, the site of your pain becomes the target. Most men who receive spot radiation report complete or at least partial pain relief after just 5 to 10 treatments.

Strontium. Pain from advanced cancer often comes from cancer that has spread to the bones. The radioactive element strontium is especially effective in relieving this kind of pain. After you receive an injection, the strontium is absorbed by your bones. Cancerous bones actually absorb more strontium than healthy bones. This directs most of the drug directly to the source of your pain. Most men feel better after a single injection.

Effects from the drug can last for several months up to a year. If you find these injections helpful, you may receive a shot about once every 6 months, at least 3 months apart. One drawback is that your urine is radioactive for the first few days after the injection, and you must dispose of it in a special hazardous-waste container. Your white blood cell count also may decrease, putting you at increased risk of an infection.

Spot radiation and strontium. Often, the most effective way to relieve localized bone pain is to combine these treatments.

Nerve stimulators. Although not widely accepted as a painkiller, the transdermal electrical nerve stimulator (TENS) offers relief for some men. Small electrodes are attached to your skin near the pain site. These electrodes are then wired to a small battery-powered unit you can clip on your belt. Gentle electrical pulses travel to the electrodes and divert your pain-sensing nerves.

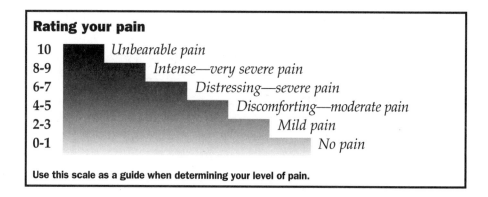

Rating your pain

10	*Unbearable pain*
8-9	*Intense—very severe pain*
6-7	*Distressing—severe pain*
4-5	*Discomforting—moderate pain*
2-3	*Mild pain*
0-1	*No pain*

Use this scale as a guide when determining your level of pain.

Nerve blocks. Specialists in anesthesiology can inject numbing analgesics into nerves at the site of your pain. This works especially well if your pain is in a specific area where nerves can be identified and targeted.

Treating general pain

If you experience pain throughout your body, try to rate it on a scale of 1 to 10, with 1 being very mild pain and 10 being the most dreadful pain you've ever experienced (see graph). This will help establish the best course of treatment.

Medications. If your pain is mild and no more bothersome than a headache, an over-the-counter pain reliever may be all that you need. If your pain is more intense, you may need a stronger prescription medication. Discuss this with your doctor.

Narcotics are commonly taken to relieve cancer pain. Some narcotics are natural compounds derived from opium. Others are synthetic medications that work in a similar manner. Narcotics include:
- butorphanol (Stadol)
- codeine (aspirin with codeine, Tylenol with codeine)
- fentanyl (Duragesic, Sublimaze)
- hydrocodone (Lorcet, Lortab, Vicodin)
- hydromorphone (Dilaudid)
- levorphanol (Levo-Dromoran)
- meperidine (Demerol)
- methadone (Dolophine)
- morphine (Duramorph, MS Contin, Roxanol)
- oxycodone (Percocet, Roxicet, Tylox)

- oxymorphone (Numorphan)
- propoxyphene (Darvon, Darvocet)

Narcotics can produce side effects including constipation, nausea and unclear thinking, but many times these effects are mild. Taking a stool softener will help relieve constipation. If you have trouble taking medications, some narcotics are available in patch form. The medication is continuously absorbed through your skin.

Another potent painkiller is the drug tramadol (Ultram). Like a narcotic, this prescription medication interferes with the transmission of pain signals. Tramadol also triggers release of natural hormones in your body that help reduce pain. Side effects are usually minor and similar to those of a narcotic.

Wide-field radiation. External beam radiation is widely dispersed throughout your body. About half the men who receive this treatment say they feel better within 2 days. This percentage rises as lingering radiation continues to attack the cancer. The down side, however, is that the treatment can cause temporary nausea and listlessness.

Complementary therapies

Some people find pain relief from therapies that don't involve the use of medication or radiation. These complementary practices can

---

Be persistent

The key to adequate pain relief is working with your doctor to find an effective treatment. If the first method doesn't work, try another. Keep trying until you find a therapy that controls your pain enough so that you can rest and be comfortable.

Many people think that pain is something they have to endure — that it can't be controlled. That's not true. Effective treatments are available. It's just a matter of finding the right one. Others worry that they may appear "weak" if they can't handle their pain on their own. This also is a misconception. Advanced prostate cancer can produce severe pain because of the way it spreads to nearby bone, including the lower spine. Your pain is not a sign of weakness.

be used in place of conventional pain treatments, but they're more commonly used in addition to medication or radiation. They range from distracting yourself with good music to the use of acupuncture. Complementary therapies are discussed in detail in Chapter 12.

Answers to your questions

Can hormone therapy control prostate cancer for several years?
Yes. Many cancers adapt and learn to grow without the presence of hormones within about 1 to 3 years. But for some men, hormone therapy can control the spread of cancer for up to 10 years.

Will hormone therapy affect my voice or outward appearance?
No. They should remain the same.

What about laser therapy? Is it used for prostate cancer?
No. Laser therapy is an effective treatment for benign prostatic hyperplasia (BPH), but is not satisfactory for prostate cancer. There's no way of knowing if the laser destroyed all of the cancer cells, or just some of them.

Do I need to worry about becoming addicted to painkillers?
Many pain medications can be used effectively over many months and years without danger of addiction. If you have cancer — especially advanced cancer — relief of your pain, not addiction, should be your primary concern.

Chapter 9

Coping with Complications

Prostate cancer is often a double blow. The first blow is learning you have cancer. The second comes when you find out that treating the cancer could possibly leave you impotent or incontinent. This can be even more difficult to accept than your cancer.

Fortunately, these side effects aren't always permanent. But even when they are, they don't have to be devastating. Therapies are available to help you manage the complications of prostate treatment, so you can continue to lead a productive life.

Learning to control incontinence

Incontinence after prostate cancer treatment is fairly uncommon, occurring in about 1 in 10 men. But when it does happen, it can be frustrating and embarrassing, and it can unavoidably change your life. You may stop exercising, quit going out, or even resist the urge to laugh because you're afraid of accidentally wetting yourself.

Like many men, you also may be too embarrassed to ask for help — only 1 out of 10 people with incontinence seeks medical advice. Or, perhaps, you think your incontinence is the price you have to pay for having cancer, and that you'll just have to learn to live with it. That's not true. Incontinence can often be successfully treated.

Identifying the problem

One of the following tests can help diagnose the type of incontinence you have and how best to treat it.

Cystogram. A dye is inserted into your urethra through a catheter. The dye helps enhance X-ray images of your lower urinary tract and identify an abnormality.

Cystometrogram. A device that's attached to a catheter measures the amount of pressure in your bladder as it fills with, and then releases, water.

Cystoscopy. A thin tube with a light and a lens is inserted into your urethra so your doctor can see how well your sphincter muscles are working.

Urinary flow rate. It measures the speed at which urine leaves the penis.

During urination, a ring of muscle around the opening at the bottom of your bladder, called the urinary sphincter, relaxes. Your bladder then contracts, pushing urine past your relaxed sphincter through your urethra. The sphincter's ability to function depends on pelvic floor muscles in your lower pelvis.

Treatments for prostate cancer — surgery, radiation or cryosurgery — can injure your pelvic floor muscles and the nerves that control them, producing incontinence. Often, though not always, the injury heals over weeks to months as the muscles slowly regain their strength and their ability to shut off your flow of urine.

Types of incontinence

Urinary incontinence is generally divided into four categories:

Stress. This is the most common type. It's caused by a burst of physical activity that puts pressure on the bladder, such as lifting a heavy object, swinging a golf club, coughing, sneezing or laughing. Your weakened sphincter muscle is unable to keep your urine in your bladder, and some leaks out.

Urge. You feel an immediate need to urinate, and you may wet yourself before you get to the bathroom. This happens when your bladder is too sensitive to the stretching that occurs as it fills with urine. It contracts prematurely, trying to expel the urine.

Overflow. Your bladder may not contract as it should, so you can't empty it when you urinate. Scar tissue at the base of the bladder or the narrowing of the urethra also can interfere with your urine flow and your ability to empty your bladder (see "What's a urethral stricture?"). The result is that urine builds up in the bladder and puts added pressure on the bladder muscles. You may experience frequent dribbling, and it may take you a long time to urinate. When you're done urinating, you may feel as if your bladder is still full. In severe cases, you can't urinate, even when you feel the need to go.

Mixed. This is a combination of two or more types of incontinence, such as stress and urge incontinence.

What's a urethral stricture?

Urethral stricture is a narrowing of the urethra that occurs in about 5 percent to 8 percent of people who have a radical prostatectomy. When your prostate is removed, the upper portion of the urethra is attached to the underside of your bladder. This helps support the urinary channel, which normally is surrounded by the prostate. Sometimes, scar tissue can develop around the area where the urethra and bladder are attached, causing the urethra to narrow.

Usually, the first line of treatment is to stretch the urethra by dilating it with a thin instrument that's inserted into the urethra. This is the simplest and safest approach.

Occasionally, the stricture needs to be opened surgically by threading a small tube and cutting tool into the urethra. In some people, these procedures must be repeated more than once because of renarrowing.

If the stricture is severe, your doctor may suggest laser treatment to vaporize scar tissue. Conventional surgery to remove the tissue is rare and is generally recommended only when other treatments have failed.

Treatments for incontinence

After surgery for prostate cancer, you'll need to use a catheter for several days while swollen tissues heal. Once the catheter is removed, you'll probably need to wear absorbent underwear. Some products are heavily padded and bulky, designed to be worn only at home or during the night. Others are briefs, which are less bulky and can be worn as underwear. There also are pads of varying thickness that you can wear inside regular cloth underwear.

Aside from protective undergarments, your doctor may suggest some of the following treatments, depending on the type of incontinence you have, its severity, and the chances that it will naturally improve over time. Most men eventually see a noticeable reduction in urine leakage. However, there may still be times, such as during vigorous exercise, when you may want the added security of absorbent underwear.

Behavior modification. This includes timed urination, that is, going to the bathroom according to the clock rather than waiting for the urge to go. You may start off urinating every hour or so and then build up to a longer, more acceptable interval. You also may need to avoid alcohol and caffeine, which cause you to urinate more. Reducing the amount of beverages you drink in the evening will help. For stress incontinence, crossing your legs during certain events — such as when you feel a sneeze coming — may prevent urine from leaking.

Pelvic floor muscle exercises. These exercises, called Kegel exercises, involve contracting and releasing your pelvic floor muscles to help improve muscle condition and tone (see "Strengthening your pelvic floor muscles").

You want to exercise two groups of muscles: the muscles that you tighten when you want to prevent a bowel movement or hold back gas, and the muscles at the base of your penis that you use to ejaculate semen or expel the final drops of urine.

As muscle tone and strength improve, you'll gain greater control over your bladder. Kegel exercises are most effective for mild to moderate incontinence and often bring considerable improvement in about 12 weeks.

Strengthening your pelvic floor muscles

It's generally best to do Kegel exercises just once or twice a day. Performing them too often may make your muscles tired and cause more leakage. Follow these steps:

1. Tighten those muscles you use to stop a bowel movement.
2. At the same time, tighten the muscles at the base of your penis. (You may feel your penis pull in slightly toward your body.)
3. Hold both sets of muscles as tightly as possible for a count of 5.
4. Relax your muscles and rest for 1 minute.
5. Repeat this exercise six times.

When you're able to do the exercises easily, increase the number of repetitions to 10 and decrease the rest period between repetitions to 10 seconds. Also, try to do the exercises in different positions — while standing, sitting and lying down. Some men find it helpful to do the exercises while sitting on the toilet seat. You might also consider doing them before going to bed. This allows your muscles to rest while you sleep.

If you have problems doing Kegel exercises, a physical therapist may be able to help you with the use of biofeedback or electrical stimulation. In biofeedback, electrodes that monitor muscle contractions are placed on your skin near your pelvic muscles. They record the strength of the contractions and allow you to see if you're using the right muscles. Electrical stimulation involves using mild electrical impulses to stimulate your pelvic floor muscles to contract.

Medications. Drugs such as hyoscyamine (Cystospaz, Urised), oxybutynin (Ditropan), and tolterodine (Detrol) help control urge incontinence by relaxing abdominal muscles and decreasing bladder contractions. You generally take the medication two to four times a day, depending on how well you can tolerate it. Side effects may include dry mouth, blurred vision and constipation.

The decongestant pseudoephedrine, used in many over-the-counter allergy and cold medications, is sometimes recommended for stress incontinence. It slightly tightens the urinary sphincter, reducing leakage during episodes of pressure. However, pseudoephedrine can produce a rapid heartbeat in some people. Even though the medication is available without prescription, you shouldn't use it regularly without first consulting your doctor.

Catheters. If your bladder can't contract forcefully enough to expel urine, you may need to practice self-catheterization. You're taught by your doctor or a nurse how to insert a soft, narrow tube (catheter) inside your penis and thread it into your bladder. You do this procedure every 4 to 6 hours. Though this sounds difficult and painful, after a few times most men lose their anxiety about the procedure and are comfortable doing it. You can carry the catheter with you. All you need is the privacy of a restroom.

Another type of catheter is a condom catheter, worn over the penis. The condom contains a tube that drains urine from the condom into an attached leg bag that you wear. These devices generally aren't recommended because they can cause infection.

Penile clamps. This device clamps onto the outside of your penis, squeezing the urethra closed to prevent leakage. Clamps aren't advised because they can scar or damage the penis.

Surgery. If you've had leakage problems for at least a year without any sign of improvement from medicine or exercises, your doctor may suggest surgery. Several surgical procedures are available:

Bulking agents. The least invasive procedure involves injecting a bulking substance into the lining of your urethra at the base of your bladder to reduce leakage. The most common bulking agent is collagen, a protein found naturally in your body. The collagen used in surgery comes from cows.

During this procedure, a tube that contains a light and a lens (cystoscope) is inserted into your penis and up to the bottom of your bladder. A needle containing the bulking substance is then threaded through the tube. When the needle reaches the base of your bladder, the doctor injects the bulking substance into surrounding urethral tissues, where it puffs up the tissues and narrows the opening of your bladder.

You may need three or four injections before you notice an improvement in your bladder control. And because your body absorbs collagen, you'll probably need repeated injections. The procedure provides complete bladder control in about 30 percent of men and partial improvement for 50 percent of men.

If your incontinence is a result of radiation treatment, you may not be a good candidate for this procedure, because tough scar tissue caused by the radiation can prevent the bulking agent from working properly.

Artificial sphincter. The most effective treatment for severe, long-term incontinence is to implant a device called an artificial sphincter that functions like your natural sphincter. The device is an inflatable silicone cuff that's placed around the urethra or the base of your bladder.

The cuff operates a little like an arm cuff for taking blood pressure, except that it's much smaller. Instead of inflating with air, it inflates with a saline solution that's stored in a tiny reservoir in your lower abdomen. You inflate the cuff by triggering a pump implanted in your scrotum. The cuff squeezes, shutting off the flow of urine. To urinate, you deflate the cuff, allowing urine to flow out of your bladder.

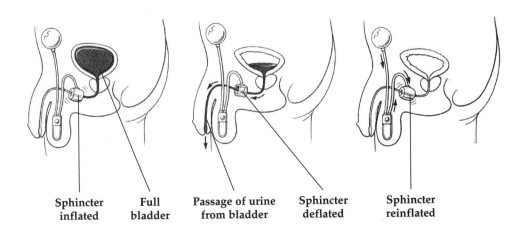

| Sphincter inflated | Full bladder | Passage of urine from bladder | Sphincter deflated | Sphincter reinflated |

An artificial sphincter uses a tiny silicone cuff placed around the urethra to treat incontinence. When inflated, the cuff squeezes the urethra, preventing urine from leaking. To urinate, you deflate the cuff, allowing urine to pass.

Most people remain in the hospital for 1 or 2 days following surgery. You can't use the sphincter for about 6 weeks, until your urethra and bladder have had time to heal. You can damage the sphincter by sitting on a bicycle, for instance, or a horse, unless you use a specialized seat.

One long-term study shows that artificial sphincters have a 95 percent success rate over a 9-year period.

Electric stimulator. A stimulator that's implanted in your spine sends tiny electric impulses to the nerves that control your bladder. These impulses may help reduce involuntary bladder contractions that cause urge incontinence.

Other procedures. Sometimes it's necessary to surgically remove blockages in your urinary tract, improve the position of your bladder neck, or add support to weakened pelvic muscles.

Getting help for impotence

Impotence can result from your cancer or your treatment. As the cancerous tumor grows, it can invade and damage the nerves attached to your prostate gland that control your erections. Cancer treatment such as surgery, radiation and cryosurgery also can damage these nerves. Although hormone therapy doesn't injure the nerves, it almost completely eliminates testosterone, leaving you with no desire for sexual activity. The nerves work, but nothing stimulates them.

There are three ways to treat impotence:

Medication
Most doctors turn first to one of the following prescription drugs:

Sildenafil. For some men, sildenafil (Viagra) produces remarkable results. Unfortunately, initial studies suggest that sildenafil doesn't work as well for impotence due to nerve damage, as it does for other causes of impotence.

Unlike most other treatments for impotence, sildenafil produces a natural instead of an artificial erection. You'll still need sexual or psychologic stimulation to get an erection. The drug helps respond to the stimulation by relaxing your smooth-muscle cells, which in turn increases blood flow and makes it easier for you to achieve and maintain an erection.

You take the blue, diamond-shaped tablet about an hour before sexual intercourse. The drug is effective for about 4 hours and shouldn't be used more than once a day. Many men are able to maintain an erection even after multiple orgasms.

You shouldn't take sildenafil if you're also using nitrates, such as nitroglycerin. Taken together, this mix of medicine can substantially lower your blood pressure and produce a fatal heart attack. Sildenafil can cause other side effects. The most common is facial flushing, which generally lasts no more than 5 to 10 minutes. You might also have a temporary mild headache or an upset stomach. Higher doses can produce short-term visual problems: a slight bluish tinge to objects, blurred vision, and increased light sensitivity. These effects subside a few hours after taking the drug.

Alprostadil. This medication is a synthetic version of the hormone prostaglandin E. Like sildenafil, it helps relax smooth muscle tissue in the penis, which enhances blood flow and causes an erection. Sometimes, alprostadil is combined with other vasodilator medications to improve its effects. Instead of taken as a pill, alprostadil is delivered one of two ways:

Self-intraurethral therapy. Using a disposable applicator, you insert a tiny suppository — about half the size of a grain of rice — into the tip of your penis. The trade name of this suppository is MUSE.

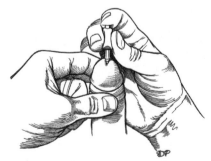

Self-intraurethral therapy involves injecting a tiny suppository into the tip of your penis to help relax smooth-muscle tissue and increase blood flow to the penis.

The suppository, placed about 2 inches into your urethra, is absorbed by erectile tissue in your penis, increasing the blood flow that causes an erection. A rubber ring placed around the base of your penis before the suppository is inserted helps trap the blood and maintain an erection.

Side effects may include some pain, dizziness and formation of hard, fibrous tissue. After a test dose in the doctor's office, you learn to do the procedure yourself.

Self-injection. You use a fine needle to inject alprostadil into the base or side of your penis. The medication needs to go into one of the two cylindrical, spongelike structures that run the length of your penis on each side. Alprostadil increases blood flow into the structures, producing an erection.

It generally takes 5 to 20 minutes for the drug to work, with the erection lasting about an hour. Because the needle used is so thin — like needles used for diabetes and allergies — pain from the injection is usually minor.

You'll need to be careful to inject the needle along the side of your penis and not at the top or the bottom. At the top are arteries, veins and nerves, and at the bottom is the urethra. If you hit either area, you won't get an erection and you'll need to wait at least 24 hours before you can use the medication again. If this happens more than once, you should contact your doctor for more instruction.

Side effects may include bleeding from the injection, and on rare occasions, a prolonged, painful erection (priapism). To minimize the risk of a prolonged erection, it's important that you test the

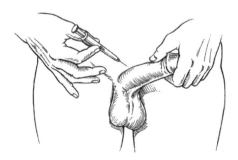

Self-injection therapy involves injecting medication directly into a specific area of the penis to increase blood flow and cause an erection.

medication to determine the proper dose. If an erection continues for more than 4 hours, the blood trapped inside your penis becomes thick because of oxygen loss. This can damage tissue in your penis. Should you experience a prolonged erection, placing a towel-covered ice pack on the penis usually stops the erection. Taking an over-the-counter decongestant that causes your blood vessels to shrink also may relieve the condition.

If these methods don't help and the erection continues for longer than 4 hours, call your doctor or go to an emergency room. Next time, you may need to decrease the amount of medication to shorten the duration of the erection.

Other side effects, which also are rare, may include a lump (fibrosis) where you inject the drug. It usually goes away when you stop the injections. One way to prevent fibrosis is to vary the injection site and to limit the injections to two or three times a week. Bruising of your skin also can occur if you accidentally nick a small blood vessel with the needle. To minimize bruising, keep pressure on the injection site for 3 to 5 minutes after the injection.

Vacuum devices

This method uses vacuum pressure to draw blood into your penis. You place a plastic tube over your penis. Using a hand pump, you draw the air out of the plastic tube. As you do this, blood is pulled into the tissue of your penis, producing a strong erection. You then slip off an elastic ring mounted on the base of the plastic tube, pulling it onto the base of your penis. The ring traps the blood

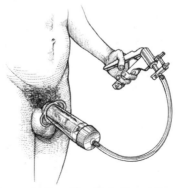

A vacuum device uses a hand pump to draw blood into the penis and create an erection. An elastic ring placed at the base of the penis keeps it erect.

inside your penis, allowing you to keep your erection once the tube is removed. You should remove the ring within 30 minutes to restore normal blood flow to your penis. If you don't, you could damage penile tissue.

Some men find the elastic ring uncomfortable and believe that it looks unnatural. In addition, your penis may feel cold because there's no blood circulation. However, a vacuum pump works in more than 90 percent of cases and doesn't require medication or surgery.

Penile implants

If previous treatments fail or don't work well, another option to consider is a surgical implant. There are four types:

Semirigid, bendable rod. This is the easiest implant to use and the least likely to malfunction. Two hard, but flexible, rods made of wires and covered with silicone or polyurethane are placed inside your penis. They give you a permanent erection. You bend your penis down toward your body to hide the erection, and bend it up to have sexual intercourse.

Though it looks unnatural and takes some getting used to, this implant requires less surgical time than other implants. It has no mechanical parts to break, and it has a high success rate.

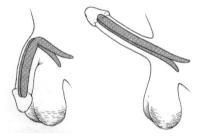

With a semirigid implant, the penis is always erect. To hide the erection, the implanted rods are bent down.

Inflatable implant with pump. This implant works more naturally than the semirigid rods: Instead of having a permanent erection, you produce an erection only when you want one.

Two hollow cylinders are placed into your penis. These cylinders are connected to a tiny pump in your scrotum and to

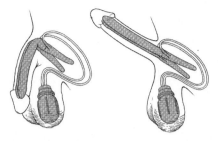

Inflatable implants include a tiny pump and a reservoir. To achieve an erection, you squeeze the pump, which causes fluid from the reservoir to fill inflatable cylinders in the penis and produce an erection.

a reservoir in either your scrotum or your lower abdomen. When you squeeze the pump, fluid from the reservoir fills the cylinders and produces an erection.

This gives you the most natural erection of any implant. It's also the only implant that achieves the full girth of your natural erection. In addition, the device is easily concealed and very effective, but it's more likely than most other implants to suffer mechanical failure.

Inflatable implant without pump. A device near the head of your penis controls the flow of fluid inside the cylinders. To get an erection, you squeeze the head of your penis. This releases fluid in the cylinders. To shift the fluid back into place and produce a limp penis, you bend the implant and press a release valve.

Interlocking blocks. This is similar to the semirigid implant, except that you have implanted a series of small blocks connected by a steel cable. The penis doesn't become erect until you lock the blocks in place. It's simple to use and easy to conceal, and produces an erection only when you want one.

Dealing with bowel disorders

Approximately 10 percent to 20 percent of men who receive radiation treatment for prostate cancer experience gastrointestinal problems. These may include blood in the stool, constipation, cramps, rectal discharge, diarrhea, or a sense of having to use the bathroom immediately.

Although external beam radiation therapy is accurate in targeting the cancer, it's often impossible to shield your lower intestines or rectum from the radiation because of their close proximity. Surgery also can cause rectal injury. However, this is rare, happening less than 1 percent of the time. If there is an injury, it's usually repaired during the surgery with no permanent damage.

Bowel disorders can continue for several months after treatment. Most improve on their own.

Blood in the stool

Radiation therapy can injure the lining of your rectum. One result may be abnormal growth of tiny blood vessels near the surface that bleed easily. Sometimes the bleeding can continue for years.

Treatment depends on the severity of the bleeding. Often, the first step is to monitor the bleeding to see if you're passing only small amounts of blood. If the bleeding is moderate to heavy, your doctor may prescribe stool softeners or medicated enemas to reduce pressure on your rectal lining as stool passes. For severe cases, laser therapy can often destroy the vessels causing the bleeding.

Diarrhea

Diarrhea can result from radiation or medication. Generally, its effects are only temporary. Over-the-counter medications, such as Imodium, Pepto-Bismol or Kaopectate, should help reduce your symptoms.

To prevent dehydration during episodes of diarrhea, drink at least 8 glasses of clear liquids a day, including water or clear sodas. Avoid dairy products, caffeine, and fatty or highly seasoned foods, which can prolong diarrhea. Signs of dehydration include excessive thirst, dry mouth, weakness, dark-colored urine, and little or no urination.

Constipation

Medications and radiation may reduce the normal activity of your bowels. When this happens, fecal material becomes packed and hard, producing cramps and constipation. In some instances, you can relieve constipation by following a regular eating schedule and including high-fiber foods, such as whole-grain cereals and breads, fresh vegetables and fresh fruits. Add these to your diet gradually to avoid possible discomfort caused by gas. Daily exercise and drinking plenty of fluids also will help reduce constipation.

You may want to try a natural fiber supplement such as Metamucil, Fiberall or Citrucel. It should help within 1 to 3 days. Fiber supplements are generally safe, but because they're so absorbent, make sure to take them with plenty of water. Otherwise, they can become constipating — the opposite of what you want them to do.

If these measures don't help, ask your doctor about use of a stool softener or a laxative. There are several types:

Stool softeners. These are the most gentle products. They're sold over the counter under a variety of brand names, including Colace, Correctol Stool Softener and Surfak. Mineral oil should not be taken as a stool softener because it can block absorption of key vitamins.

Saline laxatives. This includes the over-the-counter product Phillips' Milk of Magnesia, which works by increasing water content in your stool.

Stimulant laxatives. These are the most powerful and should be taken only when other measures fail to induce a bowel movement. Over-the-counter brand names include Dulcolax, Ex-Lax and Senokot.

Answers to your questions

How long can I expect to wear absorbent underwear after treatment?
The length of time varies. One to 4 months isn't unusual.

What's the difference between impotence and erectile dysfunction?
The terms are often used interchangeably, but they aren't exactly the same. Impotence means that your penis is unable to become firm (erect) or stay firm long enough to have sexual intercourse. Erectile dysfunction includes impotence, plus other abnormalties, such as a prolonged erection or an abnormal curvature of the penis.

If I have good erections before treatment, does that increase the chance I'll be able to have normal erections afterward?
Yes. Younger, healthier men experiencing strong erections are far more likely to continue normal erections after treatment than older men, or men already having erectile problems.

Are treatments for incontinence and impotence covered by Medicare?
Most are. However, Medicare may not pay the entire cost, especially for medications. You may have to pay a portion of the cost yourself.

Chapter 10

Getting On with Life

There's no doubt prostate cancer can change your life. Day in and day out, it can dominate your thinking and your actions — shattering your daily routine, shredding your emotions and eroding your relationships.

But it doesn't have to. Armed with insights from health care professionals and others who have been through it, you can learn to cope with cancer and minimize its effects. There is life with and following prostate cancer, and that life can be enjoyable.

Preparing for follow-up visits

Going in for checkups is one thing many people with cancer dread. For several days before each visit you may start worrying, afraid that your doctor will find something terribly wrong. And once you get to the doctor's office, the sights, sounds and smells may dredge up memories that you'd prefer to forget.

This is natural. But try to balance these negative associations with positive ones. Keep in mind that the medical treatment you have received, and continue to receive, is good. It's helping you stay alive. Asking plenty of questions during your first few follow-up visits — such as how frequently you'll need checkups and what tests you'll receive — also can help to make later visits a little less nerve-racking.

At first, you may need to see your doctor every 3 to 4 months. Eventually, your visits may spread out to only once or twice a year. In addition to a physical exam, each checkup may include X-rays and a prostate-specific antigen (PSA) test to make sure the cancer hasn't returned or progressed. Your doctor may periodically examine you for other cancers, such as colon cancer. With early detection, many other cancers also can be cured or controlled.

Questions for your doctor

If you have questions about what to expect after treatment for prostate cancer — even if they may seem "silly" or "dumb" — discuss them with your doctor. Here are 10 basic questions to help you get you started:

1. How often will I need a checkup?
2. What will my checkups consist of, and will they always be the same?
3. What are some signs the cancer has returned or progressed?
4. How likely are these signs or symptoms to occur?
5. What changes might I see that are OK — that aren't danger signs?
6. Should I change my diet?
7. Do I need to alter my daily routine?
8. If I experience pain, what should I do?
9. What's the best way for me to get in touch with you if I have questions or concerns?
10. Is there someone else I can talk to if you aren't available?

Modified from "Facing Forward: A Guide for Cancer Survivors," National Cancer Institute, National Institutes of Health, 1992.

Overcoming cancer's emotional toll

There is no "right" way to act or feel if you have cancer. The disease produces a roller coaster of emotions that vary with each individual. What's important is that you recognize and accept your actions and emotions and find healthful ways to deal with them.

What you can expect

Here are some common feelings that accompany prostate cancer:

Disbelief. When you learn you have prostate cancer, shock may be one of the first feelings you experience. You're stunned. You can't believe this is happening. You might find yourself walking around in a dreamlike state for weeks, unable to concentrate or make decisions.

Fear. Next comes the consuming fear that accompanies acute distress. All you can think about is the cancer. You start to imagine all of the terrible things cancer might do to you. It could kill you. It could force you to live the rest of your life in agonizing pain. It could strip you of your dignity and your ability to take care of yourself. It could prevent you from doing the things you enjoy.

Anger. Once the reality sinks in that you have cancer, you may find yourself suddenly engulfed with anger over the unfairness of it all. You might even take out some of this anger on people who are trying to help you, your family, your doctor, a counselor, because they're the most available. It's certainly understandable for you to be angry, but if you allow your anger to fester, it can become as disruptive to your life as the cancer itself.

Anxiety. If you experience side effects from your treatment, such as impotence or incontinence, talking about them, as well as the cancer, can be embarrassing.

Impotence or incontinence also can undermine your self-confidence. You may withdraw from others and from social and business gatherings because you're afraid of embarrassing yourself. This can be difficult to overcome if you've always been a self-confident person.

Emptiness. If you've had surgery to remove your prostate, you may feel a void that's hard to describe, especially if the surgery has caused impotence. You might sense a loss of maleness. You may feel as though you're less of a man, just as some women may feel they're less feminine after a hysterectomy or breast removal.

Treatment for prostate cancer can reduce or eliminate production of male hormones, mainly testosterone. This can affect how you respond to daily events. It might be more difficult for you to get worked up about events that used to excite you, such as a new project at work or an outing with your close friends. This could trouble you and your family, leaving all of you worried that you've lost your zest for life.

Depression. Depression is common among people with cancer. You may grow deeply sad and discouraged over what has happened to you. You may even become pessimistic about your future. These feelings may last for only a short time, they may come and go, or they may linger for weeks or months.

Depression that lingers can interfere with your ability to manage your life. It can precipitate a downward spiral that can make you more and more miserable. Because you're depressed, you don't put any effort into coping with your daily problems. And when the problems get worse, so does your depression.

A person with depression may have some, most, or all of these symptoms:

- Lasting sadness
- Loss of interest or pleasure in most activities
- Neglect of personal responsibilities and personal care
- Irritability and mood swings
- Change in appetite, and weight gain or loss
- Recurrent morning awakenings or other changes in sleep patterns
- Feelings of restlessness
- Feelings of hopelessness or helplessness
- Extreme fatigue, loss of energy, or slowed movements
- Continuous negative view of the world and others
- Feelings of worthlessness and inappropriate feelings of guilt
- Decreased concentration, attention and memory
- Increased focus on physical complaints
- Thoughts of death or suicide

Depression should be treated. With treatment — which most often involves taking an antidepressant — up to 80 percent of people show improvement in symptoms within a matter of weeks. However, many people don't receive treatment because they're unaware of their condition or they don't view depression as a serious problem. Instead, they think that they can handle the condition on their own.

What you can do

You may not be able to get rid of your distressing feelings. But you can find positive ways to deal with them so they don't dominate your life. The following strategies can help you cope with some of the difficulties of cancer:

Be prepared. Ask your doctor questions and read about prostate cancer and its potential side effects. The fewer the surprises, the more quickly you'll adapt.

Maintain as normal a routine as you can. Don't let the cancer or side effects from treatment dominate your day. Try to follow the routine and lifestyle you had before learning of your cancer. Go back to work, take a trip, join your children or grandchildren on an outing. You need activities that give you a sense of purpose, fulfillment and meaning. But realize that to begin with, you may have some limitations. Start slowly and gradually build your level of endurance.

Try not to wallow in sad feelings. Seek diversions and plan at least one enjoyable experience every day. This might include a hobby, playing golf, or going to a movie. Make it something you enjoy and look forward to.

Get plenty of exercise. Exercise helps fight depression and is a good way to relieve tension and aggression.

Look for ways to compensate. If you have problems with incontinence, sit in the back of the movie theater or meeting room instead of the front. That way you're less conspicuous if you need to leave for the bathroom. Sit in an aisle seat on an airplane or train. Wear absorbent undergarments if you're not sure whether you'll be near a bathroom. Avoid caffeinated products that increase urination.

Open up to a friend, family member or counselor. Cancer is too heavy a load to carry all by yourself. Sometimes it helps to talk with someone about your deepest feelings and fears. Your mind and body aren't separate. The better you feel emotionally, the better you're physically able to cope with your illness.

Seek sexual contact. Your natural reaction to impotence may be to avoid all sexual contact. Don't fall for this feeling. Touching, holding, hugging and caressing may become far more important to you and your partner. In fact, the closeness you develop in these actions can produce greater sexual intimacy than you've ever had before. There are many ways to express your sexuality.

Spirituality and healing

Spiritual peace can be a powerful healing force. Spirituality is often confused with religion. But spirituality isn't so much connected to a specific belief or form of worship as it is with the spirit or the soul. Spirituality is about meaning, values and purpose in life.

Religion may be one way of expressing spirituality, but it's not the only way. For some people, spirituality is feeling in tune with nature and the universe. For others, spirituality is expressed through music, meditation or art.

Numerous studies have attempted to measure the effect of spirituality on illness and recovery. In reviewing many of these studies, researchers at Georgetown University School of Medicine found that at least 80 percent of studies suggest that spiritual beliefs have a beneficial effect on health. The researchers concluded that people who consider themselves to be spiritual enjoy better health, live longer, recover from illness more quickly and with fewer complications, suffer less depression and chemical addiction, have lower blood pressure, and cope better with serious disease, including cancer.

No one knows exactly how spirituality affects health. Some experts attribute the healing effect to hope, which is known to benefit your immune system. Others liken spiritual acts and beliefs to meditation, which decreases muscle tension and can lower your heart rate. Still others point to the social connectedness spirituality often provides.

An important point to keep in mind: Although spirituality is associated with healing and better health, it isn't a cure. Spirituality can help you live more fully despite your symptoms, but no studies have found that it actually cures health problems. It's best to view spirituality as a helpful healing force — as a supplement to, but not a substitute for, traditional medical care.

Look for the positive. Cancer doesn't have to be all negative. Good can come out of it. Confrontation with cancer may lead you to grow emotionally and spiritually, to identify what really matters to you, to settle long-standing disputes, and to spend more time with people important to you.

Regaining your strength

Fatigue is a common side effect of prostate cancer and treatment. It can be a frustrating obstacle when you're struggling to keep a normal schedule and maintain a good quality of life. Fatigue may result for any number of reasons:
- Stress and depression over your diagnosis
- Difficulty sleeping
- Surgery or radiation therapy
- Metabolic abnormalities related to the cancer or its treatment
- Low red blood cell count (anemia) from cancer or treatment

Self-care for fatigue
To help reduce fatigue, follow these steps:

Tell your doctor. Don't hide your fatigue or try to ignore it. There may be a physical cause, such as anemia, that can be treated.

Rest. Don't fight fatigue. If you need short naps during the day, take them.

Set reasonable goals. Take one day at a time and try not to overdo it. But don't sit back and do nothing, either. Inactivity also produces fatigue.

Delegate chores. You may need to ask others to do tasks you've traditionally done, such as cutting the grass or shoveling snow.

Practice relaxation techniques. Wrestling with heavy emotions, such as anxiety and fear, can contribute to your fatigue. Talk with your doctor, nurse or a counselor about stress reduction techniques, and which ones might work best for you (see "Simple ways to relax" on the following page).

Try to get a good night's sleep. Here are some suggestions that can help you sleep better:

- Get in the habit of going to bed and waking up at the same time each day. This helps program your body to follow an established sleep cycle.

Simple ways to relax

Relaxation helps relieve stress that can make it difficult for you to concentrate, sleep or recover. There are many ways to relax. Here are some techniques you can try:

Deep breathing. Deep breathing from your diaphragm is more relaxing than breathing from your chest. It also exchanges more carbon dioxide for oxygen, giving you more energy. To practice deep breathing:

1. Sit comfortably with your feet flat on the floor.
2. Loosen tight clothing around your abdomen and waist.
3. Place your hands in your lap or at your side.
4. Close your eyes if it helps you to relax.
5. Breathe in slowly through your nose while counting to 4. Allow your abdomen to expand as you breathe in.
6. Pause for a second and then exhale at a normal rate through your mouth.
7. Repeat until you feel more relaxed.

Progressive muscle relaxation. This technique involves relaxing a series of muscles one at a time. First, raise the tension level in a group of muscles, such as a leg or arm, by tightening the muscles and then slowly relaxing them. Concentrate on letting the tension go in each muscle. Then move on to the next muscle group.

Word repetition. Choose a word or phrase that is a cue for you to relax and then constantly repeat it. While repeating the word or phrase, try to breathe deeply and slowly and think of something that gives you pleasant sensations of warmth and heaviness.

Guided imagery. Lie quietly and picture yourself in a pleasant and peaceful setting. Experience the setting with all of your senses, as if you were actually there. For instance, imagine lying on the beach. Picture the beautiful blue sky, smell the salt water, hear the waves, and feel the warm breeze on your skin. The messages your brain gets helps calm and relax you.

- Develop a nightly routine before getting into bed. Perhaps it's reading a book, taking a warm bath or relaxing in front of the television. This sends messages to your body that it's almost time for bed.
- Avoid food and drinks that can disrupt your sleep. Anything with caffeine, such as coffee or chocolate, can make it more difficult for you to fall asleep. Alcoholic drinks may help you fall asleep, but they can disrupt your sleep patterns and keep you from getting the deep sleep you need.
- Try to get at least 30 minutes of physical activity daily, preferably 5 to 6 hours before you go to bed, and keep active during the day. This helps you to sleep better at night.
- During the night, close your door or create a subtle background noise, such as a fan, to drown out other noises. Keep your bedroom temperature comfortable and drink fewer beverages before bed so you won't have to get up as often during the night to urinate.

Eating better to feel better

A nutritious diet provides the fuel that lets your body maintain its strength and operate at its best. That's why a nutritious diet is especially important if you have cancer. If you don't eat enough food or the right kinds of food, your body resorts to using stored nutrients. This weakens your natural defenses against infection, a major threat for people with cancer. In addition, the better you eat, the more able you may be to handle higher doses of treatment, such as radiation therapy, improving your chances of destroying the cancer.

When you have cancer, what you should eat, and how often you should eat, is different from when you're healthy. Normally, nutrition recommendations stress eating plenty of fruits, vegetables and grains, and cutting back on fat, sugar and salt. For people with cancer, however, proper nutrition involves eating more high-calorie foods to promote strength and energy, and eating more foods that are high in protein. Protein helps repair body tissues.

Increasing calories and protein

To add more calories and protein to your diet:

Emphasize dairy products. Milk, cream, cheese and cooked eggs are good sources of calories and protein.

Eat plenty of peanut butter. Spread it on toast, bread, apple or banana slices, crackers or celery. Peanut butter is high in both calories and protein.

Choose breaded or fried meat. Beef, poultry and fish prepared this way contain more calories. Meat also is a good source of protein.

Add high-calorie toppings. Top your hot cereal with brown sugar, honey or cream. Add ice cream or whipping cream to pie, cake, gelatin and pudding. Top fruit with sugar or cream.

Drink high-calorie beverages. Good choices include milk, fruit juice, lemonade, fruit-flavored drinks, malts, floats, soft drinks, cocoa and eggnog. Water, black coffee and tea have no calories.

Stock up on nutritional drinks. These products, available as a liquid or powder, are sold under brand names such as Ensure, Sustacal, Boost and Carnation Instant Breakfast. The drinks are

---

What about all those nutrition pills?

Should I take a vitamin, mineral or herbal pill? Can it help fight my cancer? The answer to both questions, generally, is no.

People who eat well during cancer treatment are better able to cope with their disease and the side effects of treatment. However, there's no scientific evidence that a vitamin, mineral or herbal supplement can cure cancer or help you better withstand treatment.

The National Cancer Institute recommends that you get your vitamins, minerals and other nutrients from foods or beverages, not individual supplements. Too much of some vitamins or minerals can be as dangerous as too little. Large doses of some vitamins, minerals and herbs may even interfere with your cancer treatment, and keep it from working as it should. Don't take any supplements without first talking with your doctor or a registered dietitian.

high in calories and protein and they contain extra vitamins and minerals.

Nutritional drinks can be used as meal substitutes if you don't feel like eating. You also can drink them between meals to improve your diet and give you added calories, protein and other nutrients. Because the drinks need no refrigeration, you can carry them with you and have them whenever you feel hungry or thirsty. They also can be chilled.

Some people find nutritional products difficult to drink because they don't care for their flavor or texture. If this is true for you, try this simple recipe and see if it improves their appeal: Combine one can of a liquid drink with a piece of fruit or a scoop of ice cream. Blend the mixture in a blender and serve it over ice.

If you're not certain whether you could benefit from a nutritional drink, talk with your doctor or a registered dietitian.

Stimulating your appetite

Loss of appetite is common when you're ill or recovering from an illness. The nausea, vomiting, depression and fatigue that often accompany cancer treatment can make food unappealing. To improve your diet and stimulate your appetite:

Eat whenever you feel hungry. You may be used to eating three meals a day. But when you're fighting cancer, you can't afford to limit yourself to this restrictive schedule. If your appetite and taste buds seem in disarray, eating smaller meals throughout the day may work better for you. Taking just a few bites of the right food or a few sips of a nutritious drink every hour or so can help a lot. Ordinarily, people shouldn't eat at bedtime. But if you can eat something before going to bed, do it.

Prepare and freeze meals ahead of time. This allows you to have something quick and easy to fix on days when you don't feel like cooking.

Choose foods that look and smell good. Cancer treatment can change your sense of taste and smell. So if red meat is unappetizing, try other sources of protein: chicken, fish or dairy products.

Most people with cancer find soups and soft foods are the easiest to eat and digest. Experiment with lightly seasoned dishes made with milk products, eggs, poultry and pasta. These dishes are generally well tolerated.

Try new foods. Some foods you used to love may now taste bad. But the reverse may also be true. Those foods you used to avoid you may now find more appealing.

Don't force yourself to eat your favorite foods. Especially when you're nauseated, avoid those foods you like the best. Trying to eat them may leave you with a permanent distaste for these items, and you may forever link them with unpleasant side effects. Save your favorites for when you're feeling well.

Enhance the flavor. You may find food tastes bland. Try small amounts of seasoning. You can also try marinating meat in fruit juices, sweet wine, if permitted, or sauces.

Drink less with meals. Beverages are important. You should aim for 6 to 8 cups of fluids daily. But try to limit beverages at mealtimes because they can make you feel full when you're not. Instead, save them for the end of the meal.

Change the atmosphere. Eating in a different setting may stimulate your appetite. Invite a friend over, play music, light some candles, or watch a video or favorite television program.

If you still have trouble eating a few weeks after your treatment, ask your doctor for advice. A registered dietitian who specializes in helping people with cancer can devise an eating plan with you that's suited to your tastes and unique nutritional needs.

Going back to work

Having cancer doesn't mean your career is ruined or that you'll never again pull your weight at work. In fact, 8 of 10 people with cancer return to work. And surveys show that people with cancer are just as productive as other workers, and no more likely to take sick days.

Your job is an important part of your life, providing personal fulfillment, income, enjoyment and a sense of contributing to the community. It can also become a place of rehabilitation and uplifting therapy, especially if you're treated as a valuable member of the

Curbing nausea and diarrhea

Radiation, medications and anxiety all can contribute to nausea and diarrhea. Here are some practical suggestions to help you combat these conditions:

Nausea
- Stock your refrigerator and cupboards with soothing foods, such as clear sodas, soups and crackers.
- Eat something dry, such as a piece of toast or saltine crackers, right after you wake up.
- Eat salty foods rather than sweet ones.
- Avoid hot, greasy, spicy or strong-smelling foods.
- After you've eaten, sit up for 10 to 20 minutes and let your food settle.

Diarrhea
- Drink plenty of clear fluids.
- Eat small amounts of food throughout the day instead of three large meals.
- Eat foods and drink liquids that contain potassium and sodium, two important minerals often lost during diarrhea. High-sodium liquids include bouillon and broth. Foods and beverages high in potassium include bananas, peach or apricot nectar, and boiled or mashed potatoes. Sports drinks contain high levels of both sodium and potassium.
- Avoid greasy foods, foods with skins or seeds, and gas-forming vegetables, such as broccoli, cabbage or cauliflower.
- Try these foods: yogurt, cottage cheese, rice, noodles, warm cereal, smooth peanut butter and white bread, skinless chicken or turkey, and lean beef.

Note: Sometimes radiation or other cancer treatments can damage your intestines and cause lactose intolerance, a condition in which your body can't digest or absorb milk sugar (lactose). Symptoms of lactose intolerance include diarrhea, gas and cramping, which occur shortly after eating foods containing lactose. If you think your diarrhea may be related to lactose intolerance, a registered dietitian can help design a high-calorie diet that's low in lactose.

team. Many men with prostate cancer find that getting back to work helps them regain a sense of normality in their lives.

At first, you may need to make a few adjustments. But eventually you should be able to resume your regular schedule and activities. Before you return to work:

- Talk with your doctor about how much you should work. It's often best to ease back into your work schedule.
- Talk with your supervisor about adjusting your hours or duties when you first return.
- Consider how you'll respond to co-workers who may have questions about your cancer and how you're doing. Practicing what you're going to say ahead of time can make the interchange more comfortable.

Communicating with family and friends

Cancer has a way of stifling communication when you need it the most. Family members may find it difficult to come to grips with your illness, so they aren't able to talk with you about important issues. And well-meaning friends — not knowing what to say or do, and not wanting to upset you — may steer clear of conversations about your health. They may even spend less time with you.

Here are some ways you can make it easier for family and friends to give you needed support:

Accept the emotional timetable of your loved ones. You may want to talk about important issues related to your illness before some of your family and friends are ready. Interpret their body language, such as whether they make eye contact. If they aren't ready to talk, give them a little more time to adjust.

Just the opposite, if some of your loved ones are ready to talk before you are, postpone the discussion without hurting the person's feelings. For instance, you could say, "I know you care about this, and we need to make some decisions. But I'm not ready to talk about it yet. I really need a little more time."

Not all families are open and sharing. You or a family member may be very private and find it difficult to discuss feelings.

Sometimes, it's easier to open up to someone outside your immediate circle of family and friends, such as a counselor or someone else who has experienced cancer.

Call or visit family and friends. You may think it should be the other way around. And with some of your closest family and friends it will be. They'll come to you. But try to remember people you knew who were ill and how hard it was for you to think of what to say or do to help them.

Think of ways to put family and friends at ease. Ask a busy friend what projects he has going. Invite a friend who's not a great talker to help you with a chore, such as cleaning out the garage. For friends who have plenty of their own problems, ask how things are going.

Accept help from others, and don't be afraid to ask for it. There are times when it's crucial to work together. Fighting cancer is such a time. It's difficult to fight cancer alone. Many times your family and friends are waiting for clues as to how they can help. When they say, "Let me know if there's anything I can do to help," go ahead and tell them. Most family and friends are grateful to have a chance to show you, in practical ways, that they care. Often, all they need is an icebreaker invitation from you.

Getting your life in order

A common response to a diagnosis of cancer — even when the prognosis is good — is to organize your life. You may feel the need to review insurance policies, update your will, or clean out the attic and give away items you no longer need.

This is understandable. Cancer makes you think about life — what's really important, what you want to achieve, and if you should die, how you can make things easier for your family. Planning for the future is good. It can save hardship and family disagreements later on. But be prepared that your family may view your actions with concern. They may feel you've lost all hope and you're giving up. Taking a few minutes to talk with family members about what you're doing and why can help alleviate their anxiety. If you're passing on keepsakes, family members may be more willing to accept them.

Joining a support group

Not everyone needs a support group. Having family and friends may be all the support you need. But some people find it helpful to have people they can turn to outside their immediate circles.

In general, support groups fall into two main categories: those led by health care professionals, such as a psychologist or nurse, and those led by group members. Some are more educational and structured, and may include discussions on new treatments. Others emphasize emotional support and shared experiences. Some focus on one type of cancer, such as prostate cancer. Others include people with all types of cancer.

In addition, the Internet now offers online virtual support groups, in which you can converse with others and receive updates on the latest cancer treatments via your computer. Be careful, however, about the reliability of information you find with online support groups. Although they can be excellent sources of practical advice, you also can encounter less than accurate, if not potentially harmful, information. Avoid any group that promises a cure for cancer or suggests that support groups are a cure or a substitute for medical treatment. Instead, look for groups affiliated with a reputable organization, or hosted by a medical expert.

No matter how the group is set up, the goal should be the same: to help people cope and live well with cancer.

What support groups offer
Benefits of support groups include:

A sense of belonging, of fitting in. There's a special bond among people whose lives have been disrupted by the same problem. You share a sense of camaraderie. Once you experience how others accept you just as you are, you begin to feel more accepting of yourself.

People who understand what you're going through. Compassionate family, friends and doctors can sympathize with your problems, but they haven't experienced what you have.

People with cancer share many common threads. Support group members have a good idea of what you're feeling and experiencing.

Because of this, you feel freer to express your feelings without fear you'll hurt someone's feelings or be misunderstood.

Exchange of advice. You may be skeptical of some of the advice well-meaning friends give you, because they haven't had cancer. But when veteran group members talk, you know they speak with the voice of first-hand experience. They can tell you about coping techniques that have worked wonders for them and those that haven't helped.

Opportunity to make new friends. These friends can bring joy into your life as well as practical support: a listening ear when you need to talk, a chauffeur when you could use a relaxing drive, and a companion to exercise with.

Is a support group right for you?

If you answer "yes" to most of the following questions, joining a cancer support group may be a positive step for you:

- Are you comfortable sharing your feelings with others in a similar situation?
- Are you interested in hearing how others feel about their experiences?
- Could you benefit from the advice of others who have gone through cancer treatment?
- Do you enjoy being part of a group?
- Do you have helpful information or hints to share with others?
- Would reaching out to help others with cancer give you satisfaction?
- Would you feel comfortable around others who may have different ways of dealing with their cancer?
- Are you interested in learning more about cancer issues?

Modified from "Facing Forward: A Guide for Cancer Survivors," National Cancer Institute, National Institutes of Health, 1992.

When support groups aren't the answer

Support groups aren't for everyone. To gain the most benefit from a group setting, you need to find the meetings enjoyable and helpful. If you find them uncomfortable, trust your instinct and stop attending the meetings.

In addition, not all support groups are beneficial. You want to be in a group where the mood is optimistic and the message positive. Some groups that aren't carefully monitored can become a place to vent and share only negative feelings that breed on themselves. This can leave you depressed and add to your frustration.

The great disadvantage of online support groups is that you don't know who else is online with you or whether you can believe everything you read.

Coping with survival

Traditionally, a cancer survivor is someone in whom there's no evidence of active disease 5 years after treatment is complete. Despite the relief of winning the battle, survival can bring other emotional challenges.

During cancer treatment and recovery, relationships with family and friends may have centered on your illness. Learning to refocus those relationships on other matters and a future together can take a new way of thinking. Reclaiming your place in your family and circle of friends may be difficult at first. Tell others how you feel and openly address their fears and questions.

Many of the old stigmas associated with cancer still exist. For example, you may have to remind friends and coworkers that cancer isn't contagious, and that research shows cancer survivors are just as productive as people without cancer.

There are also financial realities, such as insurance. If you experience difficulties switching or obtaining insurance, find out if your state provides health insurance for people who are difficult to insure. Look into group insurance options through professional, fraternal or political organizations.

Life after cancer can sometimes mean discarding old fears and uncertainties and facing new challenges. But as you adapt to these changes, you'll undoubtedly experience a sense of recovery and control.

Finding a support group

What support group you choose may depend largely on what's available in your area. To find a group:

- Ask your doctor, nurse, or other health care professional for assistance.
- Look in your telephone book or check your newspaper for a listing of support resources.
- Contact community centers, libraries or religious organizations.
- Ask others you know who have or who had cancer.
- Contact a national cancer organization such as the American Cancer Society (800-ACS-2345) or Cancer Care Inc. (800-813-HOPE).

Most support groups are free, collect voluntary donations, or charge only modest membership dues to cover expenses.

Answers to your questions

What if, months after treatment, a PSA test produces an elevated reading? Does this mean the cancer is back?
Possibly. An elevation in your PSA level following a radical prostatectomy may indicate that you still have some prostate tissue present. This tissue may or may not be cancerous. If you still have your prostate gland, an elevated PSA level may indicate that the cancer is progressing.

How long will it take after surgery before I can exercise and take part in sporting events again?
Fatigue can linger for 3 to 6 months after surgery. Your ability to participate also depends on the event and what condition you were in before surgery. Once your incision is healed, it may be fine to do some walking, if you feel up to it. Somewhere between 3 and 6 months you may be able to jog, golf, swim or play tennis at a leisurely pace. It may be many months, however, before you can ride a bicycle or a horse. A bicycle seat or a saddle places pressure on the lower pelvis, the location of the surgery.

What's a living will?

A living will is also referred to as an advance directive. It's a legal document that states your wishes about your medical care in case of a terminal illness. For example, it states whether you want to be placed on a breathing device (ventilator) or receive a feeding tube. If you choose to prepare a living will, it's important that people in charge of your care, such as your doctor and a family member, receive copies.

Does the fear that the cancer will return ever go away?

Some people who have had successful treatment are able to get past this fear. Others aren't. But in most cases, the fear wanes as the months and years pass. No one expects you to forget you've had cancer. But your fears will become fewer and further between as you fill your mind and time with other thoughts and activities.

Part 4

Prostate Health

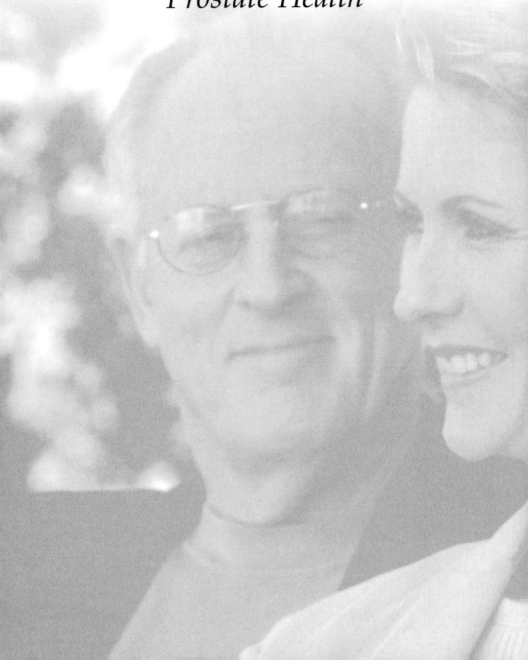

Chapter 11

Can You Prevent Prostate Disease?

A lthough common, prostate problems aren't inevitable. True, there isn't any formula that can guarantee you won't get prostate disease. But there are things you can do to reduce your risk, or possibly slow the disease's progression. The three most important steps you can take to maintain prostate health — and health in general — are to eat well, keep physically active and see your doctor regularly.

Eat more of these potential cancer fighters

The foods you put on your plate, and the beverage in your cup, may reduce your risk of prostate disease, especially cancer. Researchers are finding that certain plant-based products appear to be beneficial in preventing or controlling prostate cancer. It's not necessary that you eat these foods every day, but it may be a good idea to make these products a frequent part of your diet.

Tomatoes
They contain the chemical lycopene (LY-ko-peen) that gives them their red color. Lycopene also is thought to be a potent antioxidant, a substance that protects cells from the effects of free radicals, toxic molecules that can damage your cells.

A 5-year study of 48,000 men found that those men who ate 10 servings a week of tomato products had the lowest risk of prostate cancer. Their risk was one-third that of men eating fewer than 2 servings a week.

Lycopene found in cooked tomato products — soup, and sauces used in spaghetti and pizza — appears to provide greater cancer protection than lycopene in raw products, such as fresh tomatoes or tomato juice. One reason may be that it's easier for your body to absorb lycopene from tomatoes after they've been cooked.

Other studies suggest that lycopene may reduce your risk of colon, rectal, breast, lung and stomach cancer, as well as a heart attack. Watermelon and pink grapefruit also contain small quantities of lycopene.

Soy

Soy products come from the soybean, a legume native to northern China, now commonly grown in the United States. Certain compounds in soy (isoflavones) appear to stimulate your body's binding proteins (globulins) that keep the sex hormones testosterone and estrogen in check. When bound, the hormones exert less hormonal effect. Because prostate cancer feeds off testosterone, researchers theorize that the less effect the hormone has, the lower your risk is of cancer development and progression.

In Asia, where soy is a food staple, certain types of cancer, including prostate and breast cancer, are less common. However, it's uncertain whether soy or some other aspect of the Asian diet or lifestyle is responsible. The low incidence of prostate cancer may be related to other factors.

In addition to controlling cancer, there's some evidence soy may lower your risk of benign prostatic hyperplasia (BPH). It also may help reduce cholesterol levels.

Green tea

It contains a chemical called EGCG that's similar to substances found in vegetables and red wine. Like other cancer-fighting chemicals, EGCG appears to inhibit enzyme activity necessary for cancer growth. Mayo Clinic researchers found that even

Sources of soy

Soy isn't a common ingredient in foods, but you can find items containing soy in well-stocked grocery stores and health food stores. Here are some items to look for:

Soybeans. Soak them overnight and then cook them for 2 1/2 hours to soften. Add the beans to your favorite recipes, including soup, chili or stir fry.

Tofu. Its bland taste and spongy texture make it ideal for absorbing other flavors. Use it in place of meat. Tofu also comes in a silken consistency, which can be added to creamy soups or substituted for ingredients such as sour cream or mayonnaise.

Tempeh and miso. Both are made of fermented soybeans. Tempeh is available in a thin cake, and miso is a paste. They can be used in soups and salads, or as a meat substitute.

Textured soy protein (TSP). Available in the frozen food section, TSP looks like browned meat and can be used in casseroles or foods such as tacos. TSP also is found in soy burgers.

Soy milk. Use it in recipes or on cereal.

Soy flour. In baked goods, substitute soy flour for a portion of all-purpose flour. Place 2 tablespoons of soy flour in a 1-cup measuring cup and then fill the remainder of the cup with all-purpose flour. You also can substitute 1 tablespoon of soy flour and 1 to 2 tablespoons of water for each egg in baking recipes.

low concentrations of EGCG — the amount found in about 3 cups of green tea — were enough to inhibit cancer growth. At higher concentrations, EGCG killed cancer cells in test tubes.

More extensive testing is needed before researchers recommend that you drink 3 cups of green tea daily, or at all. Mayo Clinic researchers are studying the effects of green tea on breast cancer as well as prostate cancer.

Cruciferous vegetables

Cruciferous vegetables belong to the cabbage and mustard family, and include bok choy, broccoli, Brussels sprouts, cabbage, cauliflower, collard greens, rutabagas and turnips. These vegetables contain certain chemicals that appear to block the effects of cancer-causing substances.

Vitamins and minerals

Much of the research on the role of vitamins and minerals in preventing prostate cancer is inconclusive. Several studies have examined whether vitamins C, D, E and the mineral selenium help prevent prostate disease. Selenium, a trace element found in many foods, strengthens the antioxidant effects of vitamin E. Some studies suggest that these nutrients may reduce your risk of prostate cancer. Other studies indicate they don't provide any benefit. Current studies should provide more information on what role, if any, specific vitamins or minerals may play in keeping your prostate healthy.

Researchers also are investigating the effects of the mineral zinc on prostate health. Zinc is most abundant in meat, seafood, poultry and whole grains. The prostate gland contains more zinc than any other organ, and research suggests that too little zinc may contribute to prostate disease. In some men, taking a daily zinc supplement may shrink the prostate gland and relieve BPH symptoms. Zinc also may reduce inflammation associated with chronic prostatitis. However, it's not known yet how much zinc is appropriate, and in which men the mineral may be the most beneficial.

If you believe your diet isn't giving you all the nutrients you need, there's certainly no harm in taking a daily multivitamin and mineral supplement. However, most doctors don't recommend taking individual supplements for the sole purpose of reducing your risk of prostate disease. Not enough is known yet about the role of vitamins and minerals in preventing disease, or at what dosage they should be taken. High doses of some vitamins and minerals can be toxic.

If you have questions about the use of vitamin or mineral supplements, talk with your doctor or a registered dietitian.

Garlic

In areas of the world where people eat a great deal of garlic, there's less prostate cancer and less cancer in general. One theory is that sulfur compounds in garlic enhance immune function, helping fight off disease. Sulfur also may slow the spread of cancer cells and increase the production of enzymes that help eliminate cancer-causing substances. Using fresh garlic to enhance the flavor of meats, or adding it to vegetable-based sauces are easy ways to include more garlic in your diet.

Forgo the fat

Several studies suggest there's a strong link between a high-fat diet and development of prostate cancer. In one study, researchers at Harvard University compared the diets of approximately 50,000 men. They found that men who ate the most fat had nearly an 80 percent greater risk of prostate cancer than men who ate the least fat. Men who ate mostly red meat also had a higher risk of prostate cancer than men whose diets included fish and poultry.

One theory is that dietary fats promote cancer by stimulating abnormal cell division. In addition, some fats are susceptible to cell damage (oxidation) by free radicals.

It's still uncertain, though, whether the relationship between a high-fat diet and development of cancer is due to the total amount of fat in your diet or a specific type of fat. It's also difficult to distinguish between the effect of fat and the effect of calories. High-fat foods also tend to be high in calories.

Until some of these questions are answered, the basic message is, the less fat and the fewer calories the better.

Go for the grains, fruits and vegetables

The best way to reduce fat and calories in your diet is to eat more plant-based foods. Plant foods — fruits, vegetables and foods made from whole grains — contain beneficial vitamins, minerals, fibers

Better ways to cook

It's not difficult to prepare great-tasting foods with less fat, but it may involve rethinking your approach to cooking. Once you get used to the following low-fat cooking techniques, they'll become second nature:

- Trim the fat from meat or poultry.
- Instead of frying, prepare food by baking, broiling, roasting, steaming or poaching. Let fat drip away during cooking and drain it afterward.
- Invest in nonstick cookware so that you can brown foods without adding fat, or use a fat-free cooking spray.
- Keep on hand an array of fat-free flavor enhancers, such as broth, herbs, spices, onions, garlic or flavored vinegars.
- Substitute reduced-fat or fat-free cream cheese, sour cream and processed cheeses for their higher-fat counterparts.
- Eliminate ingredients used primarily out of habit or for appearance. Potatoes, for example, don't always need gravy.

and cancer-protective compounds called phytochemicals. By emphasizing plant foods in your diet, you limit fat and increase the consumption of healthy compounds.

Here are the recommended types and amounts of foods to eat every day:

Grains: 6 to 11 servings. Grains — cereals, breads, rice and pasta — provide a variety of nutrients and are rich in energy-filled complex carbohydrates. Despite a common misconception that breads and pasta are fattening, these foods are low in fat and calories. It's what you put on breads and pastas — spreads and sauces made from fats, oils or cheese — that add calories.

Along with vegetables and fruits, grains should form the foundation of your diet every day. Select whole grains when possible, because they contain more fiber than refined grains.

Vegetables: At least 3 servings. Vegetables are naturally low in calories and almost fat-free. They provide vitamins, minerals and fiber. They also contain phytochemicals. As with grains, it's what you add to vegetables, such as butter, oily dressings or rich sauces, that contribute calories and fat.

Fruits: At least 2 servings. Fruit in any form — fresh, dried, frozen and canned — plays an important role in eating well. Fruit has few calories and little or no fat, and it contains beneficial vitamins, minerals, phytochemicals and fiber. It also serves as a natural sweetener to other foods.

Dairy products: 2 to 3 servings. Milk, yogurt and cheese are good sources of calcium and vitamin D, which helps your body absorb calcium. They also provide protein needed to build and maintain body tissues. Dairy products can be high in fat and cholesterol, so low-fat or fat-free products are your best choices.

Poultry, seafood and meat: No more than 3 servings. These foods are rich sources of protein, with B vitamins, iron and zinc. However, because even lean varieties contain fat and cholesterol, you should limit all animal foods.

Legumes: Frequently, as alternatives to animal foods. Low in fat and with no cholesterol, legumes — beans, dried peas and lentils — are your best source of plant protein. They also provide nutrients, phytochemicals and fiber.

Fats, sweets and alcohol: Sparingly. Alcohol, fats and sugars provide calories but no nutrients. An obvious way to cut fat in your diet is to reduce the amount of pure fat — butter, margarine and vegetable oil — you add to food during cooking. Also, limit sweets, such as candy, desserts, and sugar-sweetened soft drinks.

More on phytochemicals

The term phytochemicals comes from the Greek word *phyton*, meaning plant. Phytochemicals are unlike vitamins and minerals in that they have no known nutritional value. Some phytochemicals, such as digitalis and quinine, have been used for hundreds of years as medicines. Others function as antioxidants. Only recently have phytochemicals become recognized as potentially powerful agents that may protect you against various diseases and conditions, ranging from cancer to aging.

Determining a serving

The number of servings recommended for each food group may sound like a lot of food. But serving sizes are smaller than you may think. Here are some examples of what counts as 1 serving:

Food	Serving examples
Grains	1 slice whole-wheat bread 1/2 bagel or English muffin 1/2 cup (3 oz./90 g) cooked cereal, rice or pasta 1/2 cup (1 oz./30 g) ready-to-eat cereal
Fruits and vegetables	1/4 cup (1½ oz./46 g) raisins 3/4 cup (6 fl. oz./180 mL) 100% fruit juice 1 medium apple or banana 12 grapes 1 cup (2 oz./60 g) raw leafy green vegetables 1/2 cup (3 oz./90 g) cooked vegetables 1 medium potato
Dairy products	1 cup (8 fl. oz./250 mL) low-fat or fat-free milk 1 cup (8 oz./250 g) low-fat or fat-free yogurt 1½ oz. (45 g) reduced-fat or fat-free cheese 2 cups (16 oz./500 g) low-fat or fat-free cottage cheese
Poultry, seafood, meat	2-3 oz. (60-90 g) cooked skinless poultry, seafood or lean meat
Legumes	1/2 cup (3½ oz./105 g) cooked beans, dried peas or lentils

Get and stay active

It's well known that regular exercise can help prevent a heart attack and conditions such as high blood pressure and high cholesterol. When it comes to cancer, the data aren't as clear-cut. However, studies indicate that regular exercise may reduce your cancer risk, including prostate cancer.

Exercise has been shown to strengthen your immune system, improve circulation and speed digestion — all of which may play a role in cancer prevention. Exercise also helps to prevent obesity, another potential risk factor for some cancers.

Regular exercise also may reduce your risk of BPH or minimize your symptoms. Men who are physically active usually have less severe symptoms than men who get little exercise.

Are you fit?
Approximately two-thirds of American adults don't get the recommended amount of daily exercise — 30 minutes or more of moderately intense activity.

If you sit most of the day, you're probably not fit. Other signs that you're not as fit as you should be include:

Before you get started
It's often a good idea to talk with your doctor before starting a physical activity program. If you have another health problem or you're at risk of heart disease, you may need to take some special precautions while you exercise.

It's essential that you see your doctor if you:
- Have blood pressure of 160/90 mm Hg or higher
- Have diabetes or heart, lung or kidney disease
- Are a man age 40 years or older, or a woman age 50 years or older, and haven't had a recent physical examination
- Have a family history of heart-related problems before age 55
- Are unsure of your health status
- Have previously experienced chest discomfort, shortness of breath, or dizziness during exercise or strenuous activity

- Feeling tired most of the time
- Being unable to keep up with others your age
- Avoiding physical activity because you tire quickly
- Becoming short of breath or fatigued when you walk a short distance

When you exercise, not only do you feel better, you look better. If you think of exercise as drudgery, don't. It can be fun.

How to shape up

Even if you've never exercised before in your life, it's never too late to start. You can become more physically fit by beginning a regular exercise program.

Three types of exercise can improve your health and, when combined with a healthy diet, possibly prevent prostate disease or reduce your symptoms. To receive the most benefit from your efforts, include a variety of activities in your exercise routine.

Aerobic exercise. Aerobic activities increase your breathing and heart rate, and improve the health of your circulatory system, including your heart and lungs. They also build stamina and help strengthen your immune system. Try to do at least 30 minutes of aerobic activity most, if not all, days of the week. If you can't exercise for 30 minutes at a time, aim for three 10-minute sessions.

Walking is the most common aerobic activity because it's easy, convenient and inexpensive. All you need is a good pair of walking shoes. Other aerobic exercises include:

- Bicycling
- Golfing (walking, not riding)
- Volleyball
- Hiking
- Skiing
- Tennis
- Basketball
- Dancing
- Aerobic dance
- Jogging
- Running
- Swimming

Flexibility exercises. Stretching before and after aerobic activity increases the range in which you can bend and stretch your joints, muscles and ligaments. Flexibility exercises also help prevent joint pain and injury. The stretches should be gentle and slow. Stretch only until you feel slight tension in the muscles. Continue to breathe normally while stretching.

Perceived Exertion Scale

Perceived exertion refers to the total amount of effort, physical stress and fatigue you experience during a physical activity. For the activity to be beneficial to your health, exert a "moderate" to "somewhat strong" effort. That equates to a 3 or 4 on the Perceived Exertion Scale.

0 Nothing at all	6
1 Very weak	7 Very strong
2 Weak	8
3 Moderate	9
4 Somewhat strong	10 Very, very strong
5 Strong	

Here are four stretches you can try:

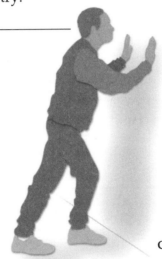

Calf stretch. Stand at arm's length from the wall. Lean your upper body into the wall. Place one leg forward with knee bent. Keep your other leg back with your knee straight and your heel down. Keeping your back straight, move your hips toward the wall until you feel a stretch. Hold for 30 seconds. Relax. Repeat with the other leg.

Calf stretch

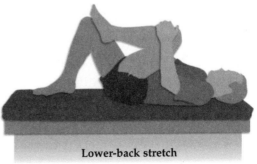

Lower-back stretch. Lie on a table or bed with your hips and knees bent and your feet flat on the surface. Pull one knee toward your shoulder with both hands. Hold for 30 seconds. Relax. Repeat with the other leg.

Lower-back stretch

Upper-thigh stretch. Lie on your back on a table or bed, with one leg and hip as near the edge as possible. Let your lower leg hang relaxed over the edge. Grasp the knee of your other leg, and pull your thigh and knee firmly toward your chest until your lower back flattens against the table or bed. Hold for 30 seconds. Relax. Repeat with the other leg.

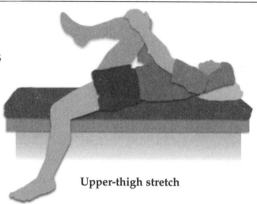

Upper-thigh stretch

Chest stretch. Clasp your hands behind your head. Pull your elbows firmly back while inhaling deeply. Hold for 30 seconds. Relax.

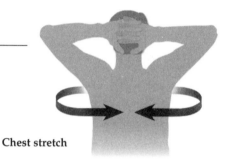

Chest stretch

Reducing the risks of exercise

Most risks of exercise stem from doing too much, too vigorously, with too little previous activity. To reduce risks:

Start out slowly. Don't overdo it. Gradually increase your time and pace. To build up to 30 minutes, start with 10 minutes, and increase your time in 5-minute increments. If you have trouble talking to a companion during your workout, you're probably pushing too hard.

Exercise regularly and moderately. Never exercise to the point of nausea, dizziness, severe shortness of breath, heart palpitations, or tightness or pain in your chest. If you experience any of these symptoms, stop exercising and get immediate medical care.

Always warm up and cool down. This reduces stress on your heart and muscles.

Strengthening exercises. They build stronger muscles to improve posture, balance and coordination. They also promote healthy bones and increase your rate of metabolism, which can help keep your weight in check. Add strengthening exercises to your routine at least twice a week. Start with 5 repetitions of each and try to build up to 25 repetitions.

Here are four strengthening exercises you can try:

Wall push-ups. Face the wall and stand far enough away so that you can place your palms on the wall and your elbows are slightly bent. Slowly bend your elbows and lean toward the wall, supporting your weight with your arms. Straighten your arms and return to your starting position. As you build strength, try standing farther away from the wall.

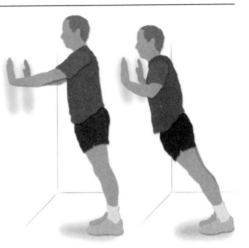

Wall push-ups

Standing squats. Stand next to a table or counter with your feet slightly more than a shoulder-width apart and your palms on the table or counter. Keeping your back straight, slowly bend your knees anywhere from 30 degrees to 60 degrees. Pause and then return to your starting position.

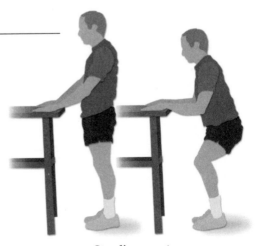

Standing squats

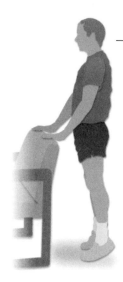

Heel raises. Stand with your feet about 12 inches apart, holding on to the back of a sturdy chair. Slowly raise your heels from the floor and stand on your tiptoes. Hold. Slowly return to the starting position.

Heel raises

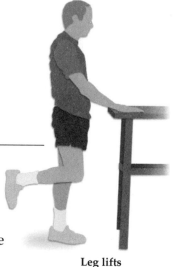

Leg lifts. Stand with your feet about 12 inches apart, holding on to a table or the back of a chair. Slowly bend one knee, lifting up your foot behind you. Hold the position, then slowly lower your leg all the way down. Repeat with the other leg.

Leg lifts

Keeping your program on track

The following tips can help you stay physically active and keep up your motivation:

Set goals. Start with simple goals and then progress to longer-range goals. People who can stay physically active for 6 months usually end up making regular activity a habit. Make your goals realistic and achievable. It's easy to get frustrated and give up on goals that are too ambitious.

Add variety. Vary what you do to prevent boredom. For example, try alternating walking and bicycling with swimming or a low-impact aerobics dance class. On days when the weather is pleasant, do your flexibility or strengthening exercises outside.

Consider joining a health club to broaden your access to different forms of physical activity.

Track your progress. Record what you do each time you exercise, how long you do it, and how you feel during and after exercising. Recording your efforts helps you work toward your goals and reminds you that you're making progress.

Reward yourself. Work on developing an internal reward that comes from feelings of accomplishment, self-esteem and control of your own behavior. After each activity session, take 2 to 5 minutes to sit down and relax. Savor the good feelings that exercise gives you and think about what you've just accomplished. This type of internal reward can help you make a long-term commitment to regular exercise.

See your doctor regularly

An annual prostate checkup can't reduce your risk of cancer, BPH or prostatitis, as perhaps a healthy diet or exercise can. But having regular checkups is crucial to staying healthy. If prostate disease does develop, a digital rectal exam or prostate-specific antigen (PSA) test often can catch the problem in its earliest stages, when it's the easiest to treat and cure. If you don't regularly see a doctor, schedule an appointment to have a physical examination, including a prostate exam, and make it a yearly habit.

If you experience prostate-related symptoms — increased urination, difficulty urinating, pain while urinating, lower pelvic and back pain, or blood in your urine or semen — have the symptoms attended to as soon as possible, even if you think "it's nothing." You don't want to risk the possibility that you could be wrong.

Answers to your questions

Does alcohol play a role in the risk of prostate disease?
There's no evidence that a moderate amount of alcohol causes prostate disease. A moderate amount of alcohol for men is two

alcoholic drinks per day. However, if you regularly drink more than a moderate amount of alcohol, it may interfere with your diet. People who drink excessive amounts of alcohol often substitute alcohol for food, and may not get adequate amounts of nutrients. A poor diet can weaken your immune system and reduce your body's natural defenses against disease.

Is soy sauce a good source of soy?
No. Soy sauce doesn't contain beneficial amounts of cancer-fighting chemicals, and it's very high in sodium. If you're sensitive to sodium, regular use of soy sauce can increase your blood pressure.

Is it true that stress can cause prostate problems?
It hasn't been proven that stress increases your risk of prostate disease, but there's some evidence that stress may play a role. Stress weakens your immune system, making it more difficult for your body to fight off disease, including cancer. Researchers also theorize that stress can produce tension in your lower pelvic muscles, affecting normal functioning of the prostate gland and, possibly, causing prostatitis.

Chapter 12

What About Complementary and Alternative Therapies?

A s Americans take a more active role in their health care, many are exploring other options for their care that fall outside the realm of traditional medicine. You may be among this growing group. Perhaps you too have purchased an herbal supplement at your local health food store. Or you may have experimented with yoga, meditation or acupuncture.

Complementary and alternative medicine covers a broad range of healing philosophies, approaches and therapies that aren't widespread in medical schools, used in hospitals, or reimbursed by health insurance companies. Although the two terms are often used synonymously, they aren't the same.

The National Center for Complementary and Alternative Medicine, a division of the National Institutes of Health, defines alternative medicine as therapies or healing approaches used as a substitute for traditional medicine. This might include seeing a homeopathic or naturopathic practitioner for your health care. Complementary medicine refers to unconventional medical practices used in addition to those treatments recommended by your doctor: for example, combining herbal supplements with diet and exercise.

The question is, do these therapies work? Some do show promise and are slowly gaining acceptance within mainstream medicine. But the benefits of many products and practices remain unproven.

Here's a look at some of the more common complementary and alternative treatments promoted for prevention or treatment of prostate disease, and cancer in general.

Dietary and herbal supplements

As anyone who has walked through a health food store can attest, the profusion of dietary supplements and herbal remedies is almost overwhelming. Literally thousands of products crowd the shelves, touting all sorts of claims.

Herbal products marketed to relieve common prostate problems, such as frequent urination or a weak urine flow, include:
- African plum (*Pygeum africanum*)
- African star grass (*Hypoxis rooperii*)
- Pumpkin seeds (*Cucurbita pepo*)
- Rye pollen (*Secale cereale*)
- Stinging nettle (*Urtica dioica* and *Urtica urens*)

Taken in small to moderate amounts, these products appear safe. However, they haven't been studied in large, long-term trials to confirm their safety or to prove they work.

An exception is the herb saw palmetto (*Serenoa repens*). Unlike other herbal supplements, it has been widely tested, and the results show promise.

Saw palmetto

Saw palmetto is made from the berries of the saw palmetto plant, found in southern Florida. Hundreds of years ago, Seminole Indians used the plant as an aphrodisiac. In recent decades, it has become a popular treatment for reducing the symptoms of benign prostatic hyperplasia (BPH). In Europe, saw palmetto is sold as a drug. In the United States, it's available in health food stores as an herbal supplement.

Saw palmetto is thought to work by preventing testosterone from breaking down into another form of the hormone associated with prostate tissue growth. In 1998, researchers with the Department of Veterans Affairs reviewed more than a dozen studies involving saw palmetto, and concluded that the herb appears to be <u>as effective as the medication finasteride</u> (Proscar), <u>and with fewer side effects</u>. However, the researchers recommended additional studies to determine the appropriate daily dosage of the supplement and its long-term effectiveness. Other studies have produced similar results.

Saw palmetto works slowly. Most men begin to see an improvement in their urinary symptoms within <u>1 to 3 months</u>. If after 3 months you haven't noticed any benefit from the product, then it may not work for you.

It appears safe to take saw palmetto indefinitely, but possible side effects from long-term use are unknown. Studies also are inconclusive as to whether some products containing saw palmetto can suppress prostate-specific antigen (PSA) levels in your blood, similar to the medication finasteride. This action can interfere with the effectiveness of the PSA test. That's why if you take saw palmetto or another herbal medicine, it's important to tell your doctor before having a PSA test, so that he or she can interpret the results accordingly.

Guidelines for using saw palmetto

Future studies should provide more information about the best use of this herbal supplement. In the meantime, the *Physicians' Desk Reference for Herbal Medicines* specifies the following guidelines if you choose to take saw palmetto:

Indications and use. It's most effective for mild to moderate symptoms of BPH. The medication relieves the symptoms, but <u>doesn't reduce prostate enlargement</u>.

Precautions and adverse reactions. There are no known health hazards or side effects when the medication is taken as recommended, although rare digestive complaints have been reported.

Daily dosage. The recommended daily amount is <u>1 to 2 grams</u> of the supplement.

Source: *Physicians' Desk Reference for Herbal Medicines*. Montvale, NJ; Medical Economics Co; 1998:1136-1137.

Cancer-fighting supplements

A few herbal and dietary products claim to help cure or prevent cancer. There's no scientific evidence that these products work, and some may be dangerous. Three popular cancer-fighting supplements are:

Chaparral. Also known as "creosote bush" or "greasewood," chaparral (*Larrea tridentata*) comes from a desert shrub found in the southwestern United States and Mexico. American Indians first used chaparral to treat ailments from the common cold to snakebites. In recent decades, the herb has been formulated into teas, capsules and tablets, with claims it can cure a number of disorders and diseases, including cancer.

Researchers believe a chemical in chaparral called nor-dihydroguaiaretic acid (NDGA) prevents replication of cancer cells, as well as viruses and bacteria. Studies of chaparral haven't shown that the herb destroys or prevents cancer, and research suggests it can lead to irreversible liver failure.

PC-SPES. This is an herbal mixture marketed for treatment of prostate cancer containing eight herbs: chrysanthemum, isatis, licorice, *Ganoderma lucidum, Panax pseudo-ginseng, Rabdosia rubescens,* saw palmetto and scutellaria. A study of PC-SPES published in the *New England Journal of Medicine* in 1998 found that the product works like estrogen supplements. It reduces concentrations of testosterone that help fuel prostate cancer growth, and in some instances may suppress the cancer, at least temporarily. However, the product commonly produces impotence and breast tenderness. It also can cause blood clots in deep leg veins and, if taken in large amounts, can be toxic.

Another concern with this product is that it can mask progression of your cancer. It reduces PSA levels, even when the cancer is advancing. If your doctor is unaware you're taking PC-SPES, PSA test results may lead him or her to think that your cancer is under control, when it really is not.

Shark cartilage. Some researchers believe that shark cartilage contains a protein that inhibits the formation of new blood vessels within tumors, preventing cancer in sharks. Shark cartilage therapy is based on the theory that capsules containing shark cartilage will do the same in humans — stop and shrink cancerous tumors. But in limited studies, shark cartilage supplements have generally been found to be ineffective.

Cancer help or hype?

Supplements are just one form of unconventional treatment for cancer. Other pratices include:

Chelation therapy. A doctor injects a binding (chelating) agent into your bloodstream that's thought to act like a claw, eliminating lead, mercury and other potentially cancer-causing substances from your bloodstream. Another theory is that chelation improves overall circulation, increasing the amount of oxygen to your cells. Cancer is thought to grow better in the absence of oxygen.

Chelation is an approved treatment for people with heavy-metal toxicity, but there's no evidence it can treat other diseases, including cancer. The therapy also can produce significant side effects, including kidney and bone marrow damage, an irregular heart rhythm, and severe inflammation of the veins.

Macrobiotics. This healing therapy requires that you follow a specific diet, in addition to certain lifestyle practices. The diet consists of whole grains, vegetables, sea vegetables, beans and soybean-based soups. Lifestyle practices include maintaining a positive mental outlook and strong personal relationships, getting plenty of exercise, wearing natural fabrics, and cooking with utensils made from natural products, such as wood, glass or ceramic.

The philosophy behind macrobiotics is that natural foods, utensils and fabrics, combined with a positive attitude and social interconnectedness, promote health and harmony and fight disease, including cancer. However, there's no evidence macrobiotics prevents or cures cancer. The diet itself has many health benefits, including being low in fat and high in certain vitamins, minerals and phytochemcials. It is deficient in other nutrients, though, and may require supplemental nutrients to balance its shortcomings.

Among other things, it's doubtful that the capsules contain enough purified protein to have any effect. Also, your stomach and intestines may digest the protein, just as they do other proteins, so it may never get to your bloodstream to be of help. In addition to tasting bad, high doses of shark cartilage can produce nausea in some people.

Knowing the risks

Unlike the medications your doctor prescribes, the Food and Drug Administration (FDA) doesn't regulate the effectiveness of dietary and herbal products.

There also are different regulations regarding the safety of these products. With prescription drugs, the manufacturer must prove that the benefits of the drug outweigh any safety concerns before the drug is approved for sale. With dietary and herbal supplements, health officials assume the products are safe until they're proven otherwise. Only when a supplement is shown to be unsafe is it removed from the market. Because these products are not subject to the same safety procedures as prescription drugs, they can contain toxic substances that may not be listed on the label. Their dosages also can vary.

In addition, just because a product is "natural" doesn't mean it's safe. Poisonous mushrooms, for example, are natural. But when eaten, they can cause serious illness and even death.

Because it's not always easy to tell which products may be unsafe or a waste of your money, the best advice is to talk with your doctor before taking any dietary or herbal product.

Mind and body therapies

These practices are based on the interrelationship of the mind and body, and the power of one to affect the other. Mind and body therapies are most commonly used to relieve anxiety and stress and to promote an overall sense of well-being. There's also some evidence they may strengthen your immune system. Mind and body therapies can't cure prostate disease, but some people find the therapies helpful in coping with the emotional and physical effects of cancer.

Humor therapy

Humor therapy is based on the belief that frequent periods of laughter help distract your attention from health problems. Laughter is also a kind of analgesic. It promotes the release of chemicals that fight pain, as well as reduce depression.

Humor therapy simply involves lightening your day with some laughter. You might watch a funny movie, call a friend who makes you laugh, joke with your neighbors or co-workers, or visit a comedy club.

Hypnosis

People have been using hypnosis to promote healing since ancient times. In the past 50 years it has experienced a resurgence among some physicians, psychologists and mental health professionals.

Hypnosis produces an induced state of relaxation in which your mind stays narrowly focused and open to suggestion. No one knows yet how hypnosis works, but experts believe it alters your brain-wave patterns in much the same way as other relaxation techniques.

During a therapy session, you receive suggestions designed to help you decrease stress and anxiety and increase your ability to cope with your medical condition. Unlike situations sometimes portrayed in movies and on television, you can't be forced under hypnosis to do something you normally wouldn't want to do. Approximately 80 percent of adults can be hypnotized by a trained professional. People who don't want to feel out of control often can't be hypnotized.

Meditation

Meditation is a way to calm your mind and body, originating in religious and cultural traditions. During meditation you sit quietly and focus on nothing or on a mantra — a simple sound repeated over and over. This causes you to enter a deeply restful state that reduces your body's stress response. Your breathing slows, your muscles relax, and your brain-wave activity indicates a state of relaxation.

Regular meditation can help reduce anxiety and stress. Studies suggest it may also reduce blood pressure and possibly even promote longevity.

Although meditation may sound simple, learning to control your thoughts isn't easy. The more you practice, though, the easier it gets to concentrate without having your mind wander.

Music, dance and art therapy

These therapies include graceful dancing, art expression and performing or listening to music. In addition to their calming and soothing effect, they can help promote self-confidence and personal well-being, and may reduce symptoms of depression.

Several national organizations promote the use of music, dance and art for health and healing, with chapters set up across the country. Some medical centers also offer music, dance or art therapy programs.

Yoga

Yoga is a 5,000-year-old practice that incorporates proper breathing, movement and posture to achieve a union of mind, body and spirit. It involves completing a series of positions, during which you pay special attention to your breathing — exhaling during certain movements and inhaling with others.

Yoga may help control stress, anxiety and pain. However, to be effective, yoga requires training and regular practice.

Traditional Chinese medicine

Some complementary and alternative therapies center on the belief that natural energy forces play an important role in overall health and healing. Many of these therapies are based on ancient Chinese philosophies. There's no proof that these therapies can treat prostate disease, but they do appear to be safe, and they may provide other health benefits.

Acupressure

Acupressure, like acupuncture, stems from the Chinese belief that just below your skin are 14 invisible pathways, called meridians. Through these pathways flow *chi* (CHEE), the Chinese word for life force. When the flow of chi is interrupted, illness results.

During acupressure, a practitioner applies pressure with his or her finger to specific points on your body to restore the free flow of chi and relieve your symptoms. Research on the benefits of acupressure is inconclusive. Many people who feel they're helped by the procedure find its hands-on therapy to be relaxing and comforting.

Acupuncture

Acupuncture is one of the most studied nontraditional medical practices, and it's gaining acceptance in Western medicine for the treatment of certain conditions. A consensus statement on acupuncture released in 1998 by the National Institutes of Health states there's enough evidence to prove that acupuncture helps relieve dental pain after surgery, and nausea caused by chemotherapy, anesthesia or pregnancy. For other conditions, evidence of the procedure's benefits is less clear. However, several studies indicate that acupuncture may be effective for the relief of cancer pain.

During a typical acupuncture session, an acupuncturist inserts 1 to 10 hair-thin needles into your skin for 15 to 40 minutes. The purpose of the needles is to remove blockages and promote the free flow of chi. The acupuncturist may also manipulate the needles or apply electrical stimulation or heat to the needles. There should be little or no pain from insertion of the needles. Some people even find the procedure relaxing.

Adverse side effects from acupuncture are rare, but they can occur. Make sure your acupuncturist is trained and follows good hygienic practices, including the use of disposable needles.

Tai chi

Tai chi (TIE-chee) is a series of self-defense postures and exercises developed in China more than 1,000 years ago. No longer used to ward off enemies, tai chi has become an increasingly popular practice — especially among older adults — for strengthening muscles, improving flexibility and reducing stress.

It involves gentle, deliberate circular movements, combined with deep breathing. As you concentrate on the motions of your body, you develop a feeling of tranquility. "Moving meditation" is how people who practice tai chi sometimes describe it. Similar to other forms of Chinese medicine, it's designed to foster the free flow of chi necessary for health.

Other healing routes

These practices attempt to cure and prevent illness through different — and controversial — routes. Studies are limited on the effectiveness of the healing approaches, and their benefits generally remain unproven:

Ayurveda

This healing philosophy stems from ancient medical practices in India, and is becoming increasingly popular in the United States. Ayurveda (AH-yer-VAY-duh) is based on the principle that mind and body are one, and that the body cannot be well if the mind is troubled.

Ayurveda practitioners believe that cancer stems from emotional, spiritual and physical imbalances in life. To treat the cancer, you need to purge your body of toxic substances through bloodletting, vomiting or bowel emptying. You use diet, herbs, breathing exercises and massage to rebuild and maintain proper balance.

There's no evidence that this practice can cure disease.

Homeopathy

Homeopathic medicine uses highly diluted preparations of natural substances, typically plants and minerals, to treat symptoms of illness. Homeopathy is based on a "law of similars." Practitioners believe that if a large dose of a substance causes you to have certain symptoms when you're healthy, a small dose of the same substance can treat illnesses that produce the same symptoms.

Working from a list of nearly 2,000 substances, a homeopath selects the most appropriate remedy for your particular set of symptoms. Generally, you take only one preparation at a time, until you find one that relieves your symptoms.

Chronic and occasional conditions, such as arthritis, asthma, allergies, colds and influenza, are the main reasons people use homeopathic medicine. However, some homeopaths believe their remedies can cure all illnesses.

Scientific research hasn't been able to explain how or whether homeopathic medicines work. And because most homeopathic medicines are so diluted, many modern scientists are skeptical as to their effectiveness.

Naturopathic medicine

This form of medicine integrates traditional natural therapies, including acupuncture, manipulative therapy, herbal medicines, and nutritional therapies, with modern diagnostic sciences and standards of care. Instead of traditional medications or surgery to treat illness, naturopathic doctors rely on methods aimed at strengthening the body's natural healing ability.

To become certified, naturopathic physicians go through 4 years of medical training. Their training, however, is substantially different from that of traditional medical doctors.

Naturopathic physicians claim they can treat the same range of conditions as other doctors. However, these claims have not been scientifically proven.

How to approach nontraditional therapies

If you're considering using a complementary or alternative therapy, practice or product — or you already are — the National Center for Complementary and Alternative Medicine recommends that you follow these steps:

Research the safety and effectiveness of the product or therapy. The benefits you receive from the treatment should outweigh its risks. To find out more about a product or therapy, you can request information from the National Center for Complementary and Alternative Medicine, or visit its Web site (see page 168). You also can search the scientific literature on the product or therapy at a public or university library, or via the Internet.

Determine the expertise of the practitioner or salesperson. If you're working with a licensed practitioner, check with your local and state medical boards for information about the person's

---

Too good to be true?

The Food and Drug Administration and the National Council Against Health Fraud recommend that you watch for use of the following claims or practices. These are often warning signs of potentially fraudulent products or therapies:

- The advertisements or promotional materials include words such as "breakthrough," "magical" or "new discovery." If the product or therapy were in fact a cure, it would be widely reported in the media and your doctor would recommend its use.
- The product materials include pseudo medical jargon such as "detoxify," "purify" or "energize." Such descriptions are difficult to define and to measure.
- The manufacturer claims the product can treat a wide range of symptoms, or cure or prevent a number of diseases. No one product can do this.
- The product seems to be backed by scientific studies but references for these research studies aren't provided, are very limited, or are out of date. Manufacturers of legitimate products like to promote the results of scientific studies, not hide them.
- The product has no negative side effects, only benefits. Most medications and other therapies have some side effects.
- The manufacturer of the product accuses the government, medical profession or drug companies of suppressing important information about the helpfulness of the product. There's no reason for the government or medical profession to do so.

credentials and whether any complaints have been filed against that person. If you're buying a product from a business or its representative, check with your local or state business bureau to find out whether any complaints have been filed against the company represented.

Estimate the total cost of the treatment. Because many complementary and alternative approaches aren't covered by health insurance, it's important that you know exactly how much the treatment will cost you.

Talk with your doctor. Your doctor can help you determine if the treatment may be beneficial and if it's safe. Some complementary and alternative products or therapies may interfere with medications you're taking or adversely affect other health conditions you may have.

Don't substitute a proven treatment for an unproven one. If it has been proven that medication, surgery or other treatment recommended by your doctor can help your condition, don't replace these treatments with alternative products, practices or therapies that haven't been proven effective.

The choice is yours

Good health doesn't just happen. It generally stems from making wise choices, such as avoiding smoking, limiting alcohol use, controlling stress, and practicing safe sexual habits. Prostate health is no different.

The choices you make day in and day out can keep your prostate healthy — or help it to become healthy again. Lifestyle changes, including eating a more nutritious diet and increasing your level of physical activity, may prevent prostate disease or slow its progression. Regularly seeing your doctor and having a yearly prostate examination increase your chance of identifying prostate problems early, when they can be treated and cured. Discussing complementary and alternative therapies with your doctor reduces your risk of potentially dangerous side effects from uncertain products or practices.

The fact that you're reading this book is an important first step, and an indication that you want to make the right decisions for treating or preventing prostate disease. It's our belief and hope that the information and suggestions in this book can help you achieve and maintain prostate health, and live a longer, healthier life.

Additional Resources

Contact these organizations for more information about prostate conditions. Some groups offer free printed material or videotapes. Others have material or videos you can purchase.

American Cancer Society

1599 Clifton Road, N.E.
Atlanta, GA 30329-4251
800-ACS-2345
Web site: *www.cancer.org*

American Foundation for Urologic Disease

1128 N. Charles St.
Baltimore, MD 21201-5559
410-468-1800
Web site: *www.afud.org*

American Institute for Cancer Research

1759 R Street, N.W.
Washington, DC 20009
800-843-8114
Web site: *www.aicr.org*

American Prostate Society

7188 Ridge Road
Hanover, MD 21076
410-859-3735
Fax: 410-850-0818
Web site: *www.ameripros.org*

American Urological Association

1120 North Charles St.
Baltimore, MD 21201
410-727-1100
Web site: *www.auanet.org*

Cancer Care, Inc.

1180 Avenue of the Americas
New York, NY 10036
800-813-HOPE
Web site: *www.cancercare.org*

Cancer Research Institute

681 Fifth Avenue
New York, NY 10022
800-992-2623
Web site: *www.cancerresearch.org*

Centers for Disease Control and Prevention

1600 Clifton Road
Atlanta, GA 30333
800-311-3435
Web site: *www.cdc.gov*

Mayo Clinic Health Information

Web site: *www.MayoClinic.com*

National Association for Continence

P.O. Box 8310
Spartanburg, SC 29305-8310
800-BLADDER
Web site: *www.nafc.org*

National Cancer Institute

Public Inquiries Office
Building 31, Room 10A03
31 Center Drive, MSC 2580
Bethesda, MD 20892-2580
800-4-CANCER
Web site: *www.nci.nih.gov*

National Center for Complementary and Alternative Medicine

NCCAM Clearinghouse
P.O. Box 8218
Silver Spring, MD 20907-8218
888-644-6226
Web site: *nccam.nih.gov*

National Hospice Organization

1700 Diagonal Rd.
Suite 300
Alexandria, VA 22314
800-658-8898
Web site: *www.nho.org*

National Kidney and Urologic Disease Information Clearinghouse

Box NKUDIC
9000 Rockville Pike
Bethesda, MD 20892
301-654-4415
Web site: *www.niddk.nih.gov/health/kidney/nkudic.htm*

Sexual Function Health Council

American Foundation for Urologic Disease
1128 N. Charles St.
Baltimore, MD 21201-5559
410-468-1800
Web site: *www.afud.org*

US TOO International, Inc.

930 North York Road
Suite 50
Hinsdale, IL 60521-2993
800-808-7866
Fax: 630-323-1002
Web site: *www.ustoo.com*

Index

MAYO CLINIC ON HEALTH

Arthritis

Chronic Pain

Depression

Digestive Health

Healthy Aging

Healthy Weight

High Blood Pressure

Managing Diabetes

Prostate Health

Vision